Also available from the American Academy of Pediatrics

Caring for Your Baby and Young Child
Birth to Age 5*

Caring for Your School-Age Child
Ages 5 to 12

Caring for Your Teenager

Your Baby's First Year*

Guide to Your Child's Symptoms
Birth Through Adolescence

Guide to Your Child's Sleep
Birth Through Adolescence

Guide to Your Child's Allergies and Asthma
Breathing Easy and Bringing Up Healthy, Active Children

Guide to Your Child's Nutrition
Making Peace at the Table and Building Healthy Eating Habits for Life

New Mother's Guide to Breastfeeding*

Guide to Toilet Training*

ADHD: A Complete and Authoritative Guide

Baby & Child Health
The Essential Guide From Birth to 11 Years

Heading Home With Your Newborn
From Birth to Reality

Waking Up Dry
A Guide to Help Children Overcome Bedwetting

Immunizations & Infectious Diseases
An Informed Parent's Guide

For more information, visit www.aap.org/bookstore.

*This book is also available in Spanish.

A Parent's Guide to
Childhood Obesity
A ROAD MAP TO HEALTH

Sandra G. Hassink, MD, FAAP
Editor in Chief

American Academy of Pediatrics
DEDICATED TO THE HEALTH OF ALL CHILDREN™

American Academy of Pediatrics Department of Marketing and Publications Staff

Maureen DeRosa, MPA
Director, Department of Marketing and Publications

Mark Grimes
Director, Division of Product Development

Eileen Glasstetter, MS
Manager, Consumer Publishing

Jeffrey Mahony
Manager, Product Development

Sandi King, MS
Director, Division of Publishing and Production Services

Kate Larson
Manager, Editorial Services

Jason Crase
Editorial Specialist

Theresa Wiener
Manager, Editorial Production

Leesa Levin-Doroba
Manager, Print Production Services

Shannan Martin
Print Production Specialist

Linda J. Diamond
Manager, Art Direction and Production

Jill Ferguson
Director, Division of Marketing and Sales

Kathleen Juhl
Manager, Consumer Product Marketing and Sales

Cover design by DesignWorld
Book design by Linda J. Diamond

Library of Congress Control Number: 2005933816
ISBN-10: 1-58110-198-8
ISBN-13: 978-1-58110-198-0

The recommendations in this publication do not indicate an exclusive course of treatment or serve as a standard of medical care. Variations, taking into account individual circumstances, may be appropriate.

The persons whose photographs are depicted in this publication are professional models. They have no relation to the issues discussed. Any characters they are portraying are fictional.

CB0041
9-149/0406

1 2 3 4 5 6 7 8 9 10

Reviewers/Contributors

Editor in Chief
Sandra G. Hassink, MD, FAAP
Director, Pediatric Weight Management Clinic
AI duPont Hospital for Children
Wilmington, DE
Assistant Professor of Pediatrics
Thomas Jefferson University Medical School
Philadelphia, PA

American Academy of Pediatrics Board of Directors Reviewer
Mary P. Brown, MD, FAAP

American Academy of Pediatrics
Errol R. Alden, MD, FAAP
Executive Director/CEO

Roger F. Suchyta, MD, FAAP
Associate Executive Director

Maureen DeRosa, MPA
Director, Department of Marketing and Publications

Mark Grimes
Director, Division of Product Development

Eileen Glasstetter, MS
Manager, Consumer Publishing

Jeffrey Mahony
Manager, Product Development

Reviewers

Thanks to the reviewers from the American Academy of Pediatrics Task Force on Obesity.

Nancy F. Krebs, MD, FAAP, Cochairperson
Reginald L. Washington, MD, FAAP, Cochairperson
Jamie Calabrese, MD, FAAP
William J. Cochran, MD, FAAP
Robert E. Holmberg, Jr, MD, FAAP
Marc S. Jacobson, MD, FAAP
Ken Resnicow, PhD
Donald L. Shifrin, MD, FAAP
Howard L. Taras, MD, FAAP

Additional Reviewer

Susan Landers, MD, FAAP

Writer

Richard Trubo

Book Design

Linda J. Diamond

Copy Editor

Jason Crase

Additional Assistance

Pamela Kanda, MPH
Jeanne Lindros, MPH

To my husband Bill and my children Matthew, Stephen, and Alexa
for your love, support, and inspiration.

Please Note

The information and advice in this book apply equally to children of both sexes, except where noted. To indicate this, we have chosen to alternate between masculine and feminine pronouns throughout the book.

The American Academy of Pediatrics recognizes the diversity of lifestyles and family arrangements. Please note that this advice applies equally to parents, single-parent families, partners, spouses, grandparents, and others involved in caring for children and adolescents.

Table of Contents

Foreword

The American Academy of Pediatrics (AAP) welcomes you to the latest in its series of books for parents, *A Parent's Guide to Childhood Obesity: A Road Map to Health.*

The AAP is an organization of 60,000 primary care pediatricians, pediatric medical subspecialists, and pediatric surgical specialists dedicated to the health, safety, and well-being of infants, children, adolescents, and young adults. *A Parent's Guide to Childhood Obesity: A Road Map to Health* is part of our ongoing educational efforts to provide parents and caregivers with high-quality information on a broad spectrum of children's health issues.

What separates this book from other reference books on overweight and obesity is that under the direction of Sandra G. Hassink, MD, FAAP, pediatricians who specialize in this area have extensively reviewed it. Because medical information is constantly changing, every effort has been made to ensure that this guide contains the most up-to-date findings. We sincerely hope that *A Parent's Guide to Childhood Obesity: A Road Map to Health* will become an invaluable resource and reference for you as parent and caregiver. It should be used in concert with the counsel of your pediatrician, who will provide individual guidance and assistance related to the health of your child.

For more information on childhood obesity and other child health topics, please visit the AAP Web site at www.aap.org.

Errol R. Alden, MD, FAAP
Executive Director/CEO
American Academy of Pediatrics

Acknowledgments

I would like to gratefully acknowledge the unfailing help and support of my colleagues George Datto, MD; Cindy Salmon, MSN; Peggy Karpink, RN; Mike Goldsmith, MSW; Jessica Donze, RD; Carla Triolo, RD; Lauren Tice, RD; Jennifer Shusterman, RD; Mary Gavin, MD; and Debbie Consolini, MD, who have never wavered in their care and dedication to the children and families affected by obesity. I would also like to thank the children and families in our clinic for providing moments of joy, sharing, and inspiration as they journey toward better health.

Introduction

Are you one of the millions of parents who worry constantly about their children's weight? Have you felt helpless as your youngster gained 2, 5, or 10 extra pounds a year—one year after the next? Have you anguished when your overweight child came home from school in tears after being taunted and teased about being "fat" and "pudgy"? Are you frightened about your child's long-term health, particularly if obesity runs in the family?

If your child is overweight, she may be paying the price for consuming large portions at meals or snacking excessively on high-calorie foods. She may be spending too many hours in front of the television set and not enough time on the playground or soccer field.

Whatever the reason, many parents don't seem to know what to do to help their children lose excess weight, even though they say they'd be willing to try just about anything. They might have pleaded with their youngsters to "go outdoors and play" or "please stop raiding the cookie jar." They might have put their children on one fad diet or another or signed them up for a weight-loss summer camp, but with not much to show for it in the long run except frustration. Nothing appears to work, and they may cringe each time their children step on the scale at their pediatricians' offices.

You Can Succeed!

If you've ever gone on a diet yourself, you know how hard it is to lose weight. Being overweight is no less challenging for children. The statistics about overweight problems in youngsters (which we'll review in Chapter 1), can seem pretty daunting and disheartening.

Even so, the message of this book is simple: *You and your child can succeed.*

No, we're certainly not going to tell you that it will be easy. You probably know better than that. You and your child may have already done your best to attack the problem for months or maybe even years, and at this point, you probably feel pretty dejected. You could be thinking that your child is living an ordinary life and that her weight shouldn't be a problem. You may have asked yourself, "She's doing the same things as other kids, so why is she gaining weight?"

In this book, we're going to answer that question and many others and give you the information and skills to help your youngster adopt good nutrition and activity habits to attain a healthy weight. We'll start by describing the concept behind this book, setting the stage for what follows.

You Are Not Alone

Parents often feel guilty and blame themselves for their children's extra weight. But obesity is a problem that's bigger than one child, one parent, or one family. In the midst of our thinness-obsessed culture, there is a crisis of overweight in the United States and perhaps in your own home. It affects people of all ages. Ask your pediatrician, and you'll probably hear that there is a dramatic increase not only in the number of heavier children seen in the practice, but also in the diseases associated with overweight, including type 2 diabetes and hypertension.

Clearly, there is no need for you or your child to feel isolated in your struggle with this problem. You are not alone. True, your child may feel somewhat "different" because she weighs more than many of her schoolmates. But there are a lot of factors that contribute to your child's weight problems that are making it hard to decide what to do about them.

If it were just a matter of trying to eat less and exercise more, there would probably be far fewer overweight children. But with increasing frequency, our society appears to discourage the type of lifestyle that could contribute to normalizing weight. Some schools have cut back or even eliminated physical education programs. Too often, school vending machines are brimming with snack foods like candy and chips rather than apples and oranges. Children are spending more time indoors playing computer and video games instead of being physically active. And among parents, jam-packed schedules are forcing many of them to reduce their meal preparation time, which often results in greater reliance on higher fat and sodium convenience foods.

It's a Family Issue

Obesity tends to run in families. As we'll describe later in the book, your child is much more likely to be obese if you or your spouse (or your youngster's grandparents) are overweight.

Even so, don't blame yourself for your child's weight problems. Don't blame your spouse or your child, either. Yes, perhaps your youngster is a little too sedentary, or maybe she's eating too much, but there's no malicious intent on anyone's part. The blame game is just going to get in the way of helping your child succeed, once and for all.

At the same time, you need to be aware that there are many ways in which you and other family members can start contributing to your child's success in losing weight. Family attitudes, dynamics, and behaviors are powerful influences on your child's willingness to make healthier food choices and increase her physical activity. For example,

- You can't just *tell* your child what to eat and how much to exercise—you need to become a role model. That means getting out the door and being active yourself, perhaps along with your youngster.
- You need to help your child make good decisions about eating and being active in ways that are supportive, not critical.
- Keep only those foods in the house that fit into your youngster's nutritional plan instead of those that might sabotage it.
- Recognize whether your household uses food as comfort or your child's weight has become a source of conflict between you and your youngster.
- Eat meals together as a family whenever possible away from the television and help your youngster select appropriate portion sizes.
- Help your child and family find healthy alternatives to screen time.

To help your child succeed, you also need to be realistic about her weight. In some cases, parents simply deny that a problem even exists. They may believe that their children need plenty of calories to just grow normally. Or they'll tell their pediatricians that they're not concerned about their youngsters' weight, explaining that "everyone in our family is big-boned" or that they're only "a tad on the heavy side." But the first step is facing up to the fact that obesity exists.

The Journey to Weight Loss

Scan the diet books in your neighborhood bookstore and you'll see that most promise a quick fix for the problem of obesity. However, these claims of fast and easy changes just don't ring true. In fact, there is a common thread that ties most of these books together— namely, almost none of them work, at least not long term.

In this book, however, you won't find promises of instant results. That's just not realistic. Instead, we encourage you and your child to view weight loss as a journey. If your child has 20, 30, or 50 pounds to lose, it's not going to happen overnight. *In fact, your best chances of success are to aim for small, incremental changes in her weight-related behaviors over the long term. These small but consistent steps are the foundation on which success can be built, and they're more likely to be sustained over time.*

Think of this journey as taking a walk along a lengthy path and making gradual progress toward your destination, day by day. Yes, like every other road on which we travel, there may be occasional bumps, obstacles, and detours along the way. Almost inevitably, your child will backslide from time to time—maybe she'll binge at a party or splurge on a handful of candy bars at the neighborhood mini-mart. But the key is that the road to weight loss isn't an all-or-nothing proposition. After a setback, encourage your child to be forgiving of herself and get back on the path, headed in the right direction.

Also, remind your child that she is not alone on this journey. You, the rest of the family, and your pediatrician are there to walk with her. It's important for the entire family to be committed to this mission. As we'll discuss later, you can't tell one of your children that "these cookies are not for you—they're for the rest of the family that doesn't need to lose weight." The entire family needs to be united, and you and every other family member should be there to support your overweight child every step of the way.

How to Use This Book

In the chapters that follow, you'll find the tools for building a strong foundation that supports weight control in your child. We want you to interact with the content of this book, answering the worksheets to take to your pediatrician to determine where your child (and family) stands and making the changes we recommend. This book will be an invaluable companion as your child travels the path toward weight loss. Not only will you be able to identify your destination, but also understand exactly how you're going to get there, the checkpoints along the way, the twists and turns in the road you'll be traveling, and how to help your child stay motivated along the way.

As you'll discover, some of the key components of this program involve your child's nutrition and physical activity. The goal is for her to burn more calories than she consumes. Much of the book will also be devoted to parenting issues. For example,

- In Chapter 2, you'll find sensible, nutritional information and guidelines emphasizing balanced and nourishing meals. We'll stress a diet incorporating a variety of healthful and tasty foods. Again, you won't find a fad diet here, nor will your child feel deprived. As a parent, you won't be asked to count calories or fat grams, but only to make and help your youngster choose healthier foods that can produce changes in her weight. You'll be encouraged to make sure she consumes essential nutrients—protein, carbohydrates, fats, fiber, vitamins, and minerals. As you'll learn, there won't be any nutritional imbalance to help your child lose weight, but you do need to monitor portion sizes.

■ In Chapter 3, we'll describe the importance of encouraging your youngster to become more physically active. These days, the average child is less active—and heavier—than youngsters of any previous generation. Children are often over-scheduled with homework, tutoring, and music lessons, and thus exercise may be all but forgotten. At the same time, many children watch too much television (an average of almost 3 hours a day). That needs to change to achieve a healthy weight.

■ Chapters 4, 5, and 6 will concentrate on important parenting matters relative to childhood obesity and effective weight management. These chapters are key components of this book; in fact, they set this program apart from other weight-loss plans for children. As important as proper nutrition and physical activity are, the chances of their long-term success are limited without the sound parenting skills that we'll describe in these chapters. We'll empower you to help your child make changes that can effectively reduce her weight. You'll evaluate how food is used in your family (eg, as rewards or bribes). You'll learn how to partner with your pediatrician, extended family members, and community resources (including grandparents, schools, babysitters, and child care workers) to help ensure your child's success. And you'll learn to deal effectively with a variety of parenting challenges, from your child's emotional turmoil and weakened self-esteem to managing her weight-loss setbacks or detours that will occur from time to time.

In the later chapters of the book (beginning with Chapter 7), we'll describe the developmental stages that all children move through and the way that being overweight can affect a child at every point in her life, from infancy and the toddler years to school age and adolescence. At each stage, you and your child will be encouraged to set short-term, achievable goals. Remember, we're talking about changes that will not only help your child manage her weight today, but could also keep a serious chronic illness related to her weight from developing in adulthood. Modeling and motivating proper eating and activity today will serve her well for the rest of her life.

Where Does Your Child Stand?

Let's get a sense of your child's current weight, nutrition, and activity level and where you'd like her to be headed. Spend a few minutes completing the following assessment forms, and share them with your pediatrician.

At the next office visit, ask your pediatrician's guidance in using the growth charts and the body mass index (BMI) graphs on pages xxxi to xxxiv. They can provide a clear picture of your youngster's present status and areas that need attention. The growth charts will help you see how your child compares with her peers. Does she fall within the normal range of height and weight for her age? Most pediatricians use charts like these to evaluate your child's growth from one visit to the next.

If your child is younger than 2 years, your pediatrician will be using charts (rather than calculating BMI) to determine her risk for being overweight or obese. If your youngster's weight gain is crossing growth percentiles, this may also be a risk factor for overweight and obesity that needs the attention of you and your pediatrician.

Pediatricians consider BMI (a calculation of your child's body weight relative to her height) important when determining whether your child is overweight. You'll find the formula for calculating your child's BMI in the box on page xxx.

Keep in mind that although BMI is not a specific measure of body fat, it is closely linked with body fat calculations. Your pediatrician may also use an instrument called *skinfold calipers* to gently pinch the flesh on your child's trunk and the back of her upper arm to measure the body fat directly beneath the skin. Your pediatrician will be taking into account your child's pattern of growth, family history, body composition, and laboratory studies to determine her health risk.

What Does BMI Mean for Your Own Child?

- BMI between 85% and 95% for age: overweight
- Greater than 95% for age: obese

About the Worksheets

Take the worksheets found throughout the book with you when your child sees the pediatrician. Share this information about your goals and begin the journey to a healthy lifestyle.

Calculating Body Mass Index

Use this formula or visit www.cdc.gov to measure your child's BMI.

■ Multiply her weight (in pounds) by 703. (We'll call this A.)

■ Multiply her height (in inches) by itself. (We'll call this B.)

■ Divide A by B. This will give you her BMI score.

For example, let's say you have a 12-year-old girl. She is 5 feet 2 inches (62") and weighs 155 pounds. Multiply her weight (155 lb) by 703 (108,965); multiply her height (62") by itself (3,844); then divide the first total by the second. Your daughter's BMI (108,965 ÷ 3,844) is 28.3. As you can see on the chart below, this example daughter's BMI is greater than 95% for age.

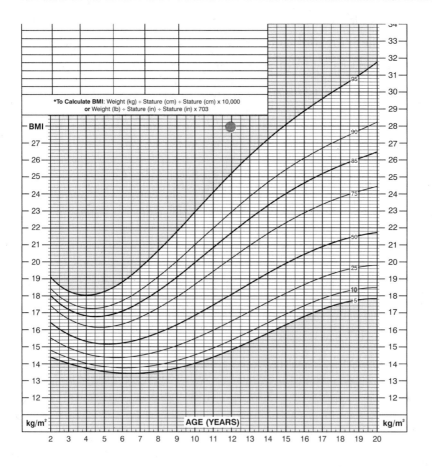

WORKSHEET TO TAKE TO YOUR PEDIATRICIAN
#1: WHERE IS YOUR CHILD TODAY?

Fill in the following information about your child. These are the kinds of numbers that your pediatrician already collects.

Age: _____   Height: _____   Weight: _____

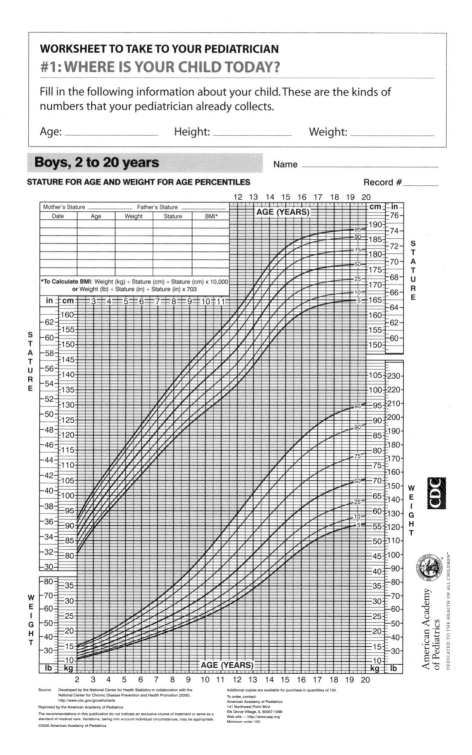

Boys, 2 to 20 years   Name _____

STATURE FOR AGE AND WEIGHT FOR AGE PERCENTILES   Record # _____

Date	Age	Weight	Stature	BMI*

*To Calculate BMI: Weight (kg) ÷ Stature (cm) ÷ Stature (cm) x 10,000
or Weight (lb) ÷ Stature (in) ÷ Stature (in) x 703

Mother's Stature _____   Father's Stature _____

Source: Developed by the National Center for Health Statistics in collaboration with the National Center for Chronic Disease Prevention and Health Promotion (2000).
http://www.cdc.gov/growthcharts

Reprinted by the American Academy of Pediatrics

The recommendations in this publication do not indicate an exclusive course of treatment or serve as a standard of medical care. Variations, taking into account individual circumstances, may be appropriate.

©2000 American Academy of Pediatrics

Additional copies are available for purchase in quantities of 100.
To order, contact:
American Academy of Pediatrics
141 Northwest Point Blvd
Elk Grove Village, IL 60007-1098
Web site — http://www.aap.org
Minimum order 100.

WORKSHEET TO TAKE TO YOUR PEDIATRICIAN
#1: WHERE IS YOUR CHILD TODAY?

Fill in the following information about your child. These are the kinds of numbers that your pediatrician already collects.

Age: _____   Height: _____   Weight: _____

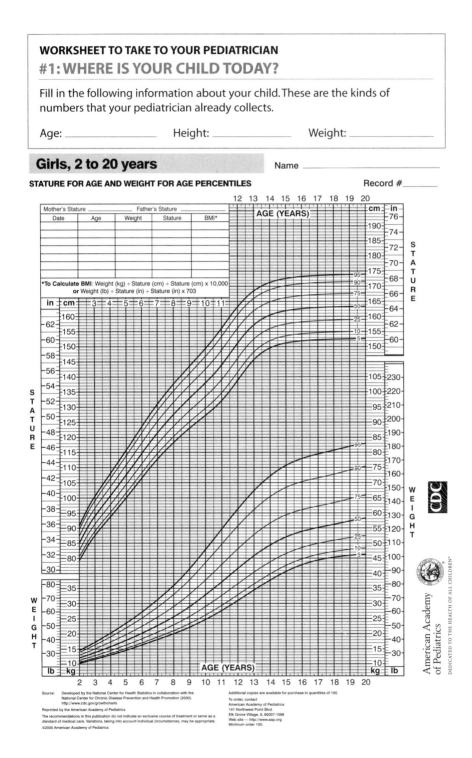

Girls, 2 to 20 years   Name _____

STATURE FOR AGE AND WEIGHT FOR AGE PERCENTILES   Record #_____

WORKSHEET TO TAKE TO YOUR PEDIATRICIAN

#1: WHERE IS YOUR CHILD TODAY?

Fill in the following information about your child. These are the kinds of numbers that your pediatrician already collects.

Age: _____   Height: _____   Weight: _____

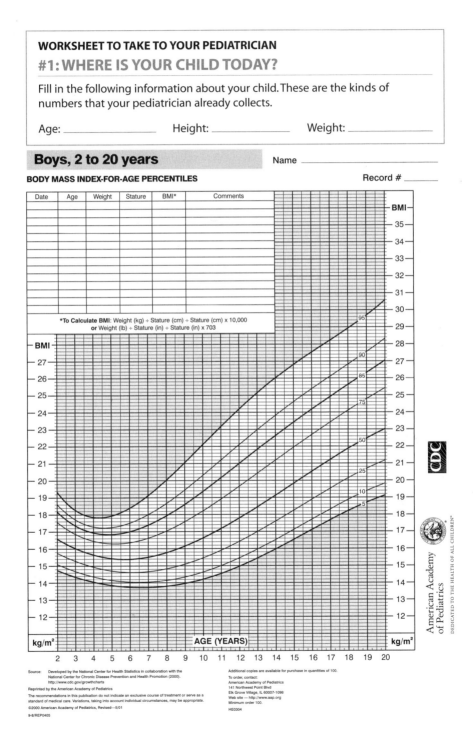

Boys, 2 to 20 years

Name _____

BODY MASS INDEX-FOR-AGE PERCENTILES

Record # _____

*To Calculate BMI: Weight (kg) ÷ Stature (cm) ÷ Stature (cm) x 10,000
or Weight (lb) ÷ Stature (in) ÷ Stature (in) x 703

WORKSHEET TO TAKE TO YOUR PEDIATRICIAN

#1: WHERE IS YOUR CHILD TODAY?

Fill in the following information about your child. These are the kinds of numbers that your pediatrician already collects.

Age: _____   Height: _____   Weight: _____

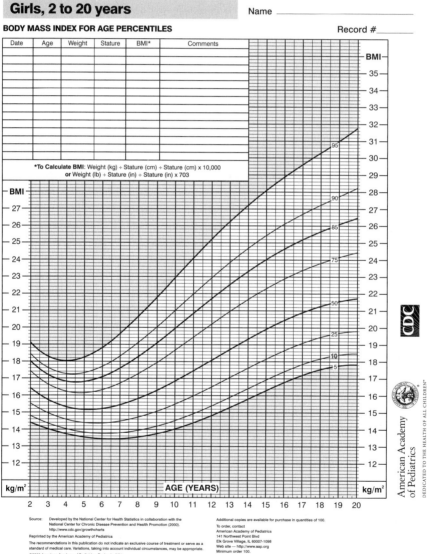

Girls, 2 to 20 years

Name _____

BODY MASS INDEX FOR AGE PERCENTILES

Record # _____

*To Calculate BMI: Weight (kg) ÷ Stature (cm) ÷ Stature (cm) x 10,000
or Weight (lb) ÷ Stature (in) ÷ Stature (in) x 703

Source: Developed by the National Center for Health Statistics in collaboration with the
National Center for Chronic Disease Prevention and Health Promotion (2000).
http://www.cdc.gov/growthcharts

Reprinted by the American Academy of Pediatrics

The recommendations in this publication do not indicate an exclusive course of treatment or serve as a
standard of medical care. Variations, taking into account individual circumstances, may be appropriate.

©2000 American Academy of Pediatrics, Revised—5/01

9-10/REP0605

Additional copies are available for purchase in quantities of 100.
To order, contact
American Academy of Pediatrics
141 Northwest Point Blvd
Elk Grove Village, IL 60007-1098
Web site — http://www.aap.org
Minimum order 100.

HE0306

WORKSHEET TO TAKE TO YOUR PEDIATRICIAN
#2: YOUR CHILD AND HIS OR HER WEIGHT

For this assessment, answer the following questions about your youngster:

How does your child feel about his or her weight? (Explain.)

_____

Does your child worry about how much he or she weighs?

_____

What kinds of things concern your child?

_____

Does your child worry about taking gym class at school?

_____

Does your child worry about keeping up with other children on the playground?

_____

Is your child concerned about being teased?

_____

Is your child worried about how he or she looks in clothes?

_____

Is your child concerned about his or her health?

_____

Other concerns:

_____

How do you feel about your child's weight?

_____

Are you concerned about your child being teased by peers? _____

Are you anxious about the short- and long-term consequences of your child's weight gain and eating behaviors?

_____

Other worries:

_____

_____

WORKSHEET TO TAKE TO YOUR PEDIATRICIAN
#3: WHERE DO YOU AND YOUR CHILD WANT TO GO?

With this worksheet, you'll begin to look toward your child's future.

What are your child's health goals relative to his or her weight (these should be health goals, rather than being related primarily to weight)?

_____

Is there a health problem associated with your child's weight that you'd like to improve or correct?

- ☐ Lower cholesterol level
- ☐ Lower blood pressure
- ☐ Improve blood sugar glucose level
- ☐ Be able to run or be physically active and keep up with friends without becoming winded so quickly

Are there eating behaviors you would like to help your child improve? (Check those that apply.)

- ☐ Overeating at meals
- ☐ Too many snacks
- ☐ Unhealthy food choices
- ☐ Eating at night
- ☐ Eating in front of TV
- ☐ Too many fast-food meals
- ☐ Very limited diet choices
- ☐ Unhealthy food choices

Are there activity behaviors you would like to help your child improve? (Check all that apply.)

- ☐ Limiting TV/computer use
- ☐ Being more motivated to be active
- ☐ Participating in more peer-group activities
- ☐ Others: _____

What are the long-term goals that you and your child have relative to your child's weight? (Check all that apply.)

- ☐ Improve your child's overall health.
- ☐ Decrease the chances that your child will be an overweight/obese adult.
- ☐ Increase your child's self-esteem.
- ☐ Reduce family conflict around food and activity.
- ☐ Decrease teasing.

WORKSHEET TO TAKE TO YOUR PEDIATRICIAN
#4: HOW WILL YOU AND YOUR CHILD GET THERE?

Let's be more specific about the goals for your youngster.

As you get started, what short-term goals do you and your child have?

_____

_____

Specifically, how does your family plan to eat healthier, meal by meal?

_____

_____

Specifically, how does your family plan to become more active, day by day?

_____

_____

What other short-term and intermediate goals do you and your child have?

_____

_____

Do you think that making behavioral changes associated with these goals will be easy or difficult?

_____

Who is going to go with you on this weight-loss journey? Who can help you and your child achieve your goals? (Check all that apply.)

☐ Other family members   ☐ School
☐ Spouse   ☐ Parent groups
☐ Siblings   ☐ Child care staff
☐ Grandparents   ☒ Your pediatrician
☐ Friends   ☐ Others

What information do you need to help you achieve these goals?
(Check those that apply.)

☐ More knowledge of proper nutrition
☐ Help with activity alternatives
☐ Skills to help your child and family make healthy changes
☐ Information about age-appropriate diet and activity
☐ Information about the health consequences of obesity

1

The Problem of Obesity

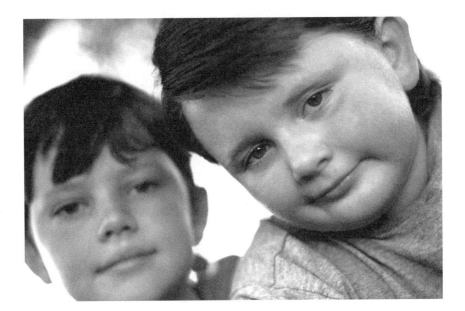

If you spend a few minutes watching children getting off a school bus, you might be surprised by what you see. Amid the expected sights and sounds of kids talking, laughing, and toting backpacks to class, you'll probably also notice that a disturbing number of these youngsters are overweight.

In fact, in every corner of the United States—from California to New York and everywhere in-between—obesity among children is at epidemic levels. Just consider the following statistics:

- Over the past 2 decades, the prevalence of children who are overweight has doubled, while the number of overweight adolescents has tripled.
- Twenty-five percent of all children aged 2 to 18 years now meet the criteria for being overweight.
- About 9 million children older than 6 years are obese.

These unsettling trends affect boys and girls. They involve children of all races, all ethnic groups, and all socioeconomic classes.

The Physical Toll: Medical Diseases and Conditions

Pediatricians are very concerned about the growing number of overweight children for a number of reasons. Not surprisingly, obesity can limit a child's physical activity on the playground and athletic field. But more worrisome, there are many health risks associated with being too heavy. For example, one recent report stated that among obese children 5 to 10 years of age, 60% already had at least one risk factor for cardiovascular disease, such as high cholesterol

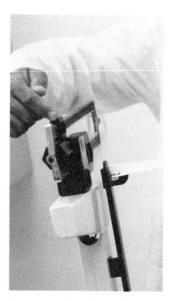

levels, high triglycerides (another type of blood fat), and high blood pressure.

Cardiovascular-related conditions aren't the only health problems associated with childhood obesity (see text box on page 5). Diabetes, for example, is another increasing concern among pediatricians and parents of overweight children. That's because a fast-growing number of newly diagnosed cases of childhood diabetes are the so-called type 2 form of the disease. Type 2 diabetes used to be called adult-onset because it almost always affected adults, but now this form of diabetes is increasingly evolving into a disease of children and teenagers, as well. In fact, recent research has shown that between 25% and 60% of newly diagnosed diabetes in children are now type 2. Particularly if your child is obese and inactive, he has an increased risk of developing this form of the disease.

To make matters worse, if your child is overweight, he is much more likely to become an overweight adult. The statistics are unsettling—about 20% of obese 4-year-olds will grow up to become obese adults. That figure rises to 80% among teenagers who are overweight. And once your child is an adult, he'll be more likely to have the same obesity-related health problems from high blood pressure to joint problems, as well as a greater risk of death as his weight increases. The bottom line is that obesity can cause a lifetime of very serious health concerns.

Your Overweight Child and the Risk of Disease

If you child or adolescent is obese or overweight, he has a higher incidence of having a number of serious medical problems, including

- High blood pressure (hypertension)
- Abnormal lipid levels
- Metabolic syndrome (A condition of insulin resistance associated with high blood pressure, high triglyceride levels, obesity, and in some cases, liver disease and menstrual irregularities in girls)
- Type 2 diabetes (once called adult-onset or non–insulin-dependent diabetes)
- Asthma
- Sleep apnea (repeated disruption of normal breathing during sleep)
- Skin infections (eg, fungi trapped in folds of skin)
- Pain in the knee, thigh, and hip (often associated with a condition called slipped capital femoral epiphysis)
- Back pain
- Liver disease
- Gallstones
- Inflammation of the pancreas (pancreatitis)
- Menstrual abnormalities (eg, irregular or missed periods, known as polycystic ovarian syndrome)
- Severe headaches with visual disturbances

One other point is important to make: Some children become so obsessed with their excess pounds and have such a distorted body image that they begin to try unusual diets, skip meals, or eliminate food groups, further adding to unhealthy eating and poor nutrition.

Rarely, some children can become so focused on their weight and body image that they may develop eating disorders such as bulimia and anorexia, all because they're trying to get their weight under control in an unhealthy way.

Environmental Factors

Your youngster's day-to-day environment—at home, at school, at friends' homes, and virtually everywhere else he spends time—can affect his risk of becoming and remaining overweight. The fast-food restaurants where he eats, TV programs he watches, and video games he plays can contribute to his likelihood of developing obesity.

For example, the risk of being overweight is more than $4^1/_2$ times greater for children who watch more than 5 hours of TV a day, compared with children who watch no more than 2 hours a day. That's because children are not only inactive while watching television, but they also tend to snack at the same time, often eating high-fat foods like cookies or potato chips rather than an apple or a pear. Even so, except for sleeping, most US children spend more time (outside of school hours) watching TV than participating in any other activity.

Obesity's Emotional Toll

You've heard the stories about the happy fat person, right? Well, as comforting as they might be, particularly if your own child is heavy, they may be more myth than reality in most children's lives. Not only are there health costs associated with childhood obesity, but your child's weight problem is also intimately entangled in his emotional world.

For overweight children as well as their parents, living with excess pounds can be heartbreaking. In its own way, the social stigma attached to being overweight can be as damaging to a child as the physical diseases and conditions that often accompany obesity. You can probably see it in the eyes and hear it in the words of your own overweight child. In a society that puts a premium on thinness, studies show that children as young as 6 years may associate negative stereotypes with excess weight and believe that a heavy child is simply less likable.

True, some overweight children are very popular with their classmates, feel good about themselves, and have plenty of self-confidence. But in general, if your child is obese, he is more likely to have low self-esteem than his thinner peers. His weak self-esteem can translate into feelings of shame about his body, and his lack of self-confidence can lead to poorer academic performance at school.

You probably don't need a detailed description of how difficult the day-to-day life of overweight children can sometimes be. These youngsters may be told by classmates (and even adults) that being heavy is their own fault. They might be called names. They could be subjected to teasing and bullying. Their former friends may avoid them, and they may also have trouble making new friends. They could be the last one chosen when teams are selected in physical education classes.

With all of this turmoil in an overweight child's life, he may feel as though he doesn't belong or fit in anywhere. He may see himself as different and an outcast. He'll often feel lonely and is less likely than his peers to describe himself as popular or cool. And when this scenario becomes ingrained as part of his life—month after month, year after year—he can become sad and clinically depressed and withdraw into himself.

In an ironic twist, some overweight children like these might seek emotional comfort in food, adding even more calories to their plates at the same time that their pediatricians and parents are urging them to eat less. Add to that the other emotional peaks and valleys of life, including the stress of moving to a new community, difficulties in school, or the death of a parent or a divorce, and some children routinely overindulge in food.

There are other obesity-related repercussions that continue well into adolescence and beyond. Heavy teenagers and adults might face discrimination based solely on their weight. Some research suggests that they are less likely to be accepted for admission by a prestigious university. They may also have a reduced chance of landing good

Your Child's Genetics

Because obesity runs in families, you need to determine just how prevalent it has been in your own family over generations. The following statistics are for young children and indicate the importance of genetics and family lifestyle in a youngster's risk of becoming overweight:

- If one parent is obese, a child has a threefold greater risk of developing obesity than a child whose parents are both of average weight.
- If both parents are obese, the child's risk rises by more than tenfold.
- For a child younger than 3 years, the presence of obesity in his parents is a stronger predictor of whether he will become obese in adulthood than his own current weight.

jobs than their thinner peers. Overweight women have a decreased likelihood of dating or finding a marriage partner. In short, when heavy children become heavy adults, they tend to earn less money and marry less often than their friends who are of average weight.

Childhood Obesity: What Are the Common Misconceptions?

Everyone, it seems, has an opinion about obesity. Some may insist that they know what causes it. Or they might have a dozen or more suggestions on how to conquer it. Yet even though it seems that our culture is obsessed with diets and a belief that you can never be too thin, there are more than enough myths and misunderstandings about childhood weight to go around. Unfortunately, some of this misinformation can get in the way of your child succeeding in his own weight-loss efforts.

To help you and your youngster get on the right path toward normalizing his weight, let's separate fiction from facts. See if you believe in any of the following misconceptions, and then read what the truth about them really is:

"My child and I deserve the blame for his weight problem." Not true. Thanks to the media and many high-profile diet gurus, many overweight children and adults believe that obesity occurs in people who are self-indulgent or weak-willed. With those kinds of attitudes so prevalent, no wonder that there's so little empathy and support for individuals who need to lose weight. However, the facts are that *no one* is to blame for your child's obesity. Children gain excess weight for a variety of reasons. Some have a tendency to be obese because it runs in their families. Others may not make the best selections of foods or portion sizes, often because healthier choices aren't available or perhaps because their parents or grandparents put too much food on their plates. Throughout this book, you'll find descriptions of other culprits and contributors to your child's weight problem that should remove self-blame. Once you understand the causes of obesity a little better, you and your child will be able to manage his obesity more effectively and realistically.

"My child's weight problem needs a quick fix." Yes, you and your youngster may wish for an instantaneous solution for losing his excess pounds, and there are plenty of diets in bookstores that promise fast results. But let's face it—there are no easy answers to weight problems (or to most other things in life). Obesity is not a problem that can be resolved overnight or even in a few weeks. (If you've ever tried to lose weight yourself and keep it off, you know that's the case.) In fact, some of the most popular quick fixes, from diet pills to herbal teas, may be hazardous to your child's health. Many of the "natural" supplements that teenagers might be attracted to, as well as the near-starvation diets that are promoted in newspaper ads and popular magazine articles, are risky and in some cases, even potentially deadly. Where should you turn instead? Working with your child's pediatrician and using plans and programs like the one in this book that are based on credible, scientific evidence offers the best chance for safe and long-term weight-loss success.

"My overweight child will 'grow into' the excess pounds that he has." Youngsters normally gain weight throughout childhood. It's a necessary part of the growth process. But some parents tell their pediatricians that their overweight children will outgrow their weight problems. However, that's not something you can count on. In fact, depending on your child's eating habits and activity level, he is just as likely to continue to gain weight, not lose it, as he grows. Don't depend on routine growth spurts to compensate for his weight problem.

"My child may seem overweight according to the growth charts, but our entire family is 'big boned.' So I don't think he has a weight problem at all." Pediatricians often hear parents say, "We're not worried about our child's weight. Everyone in our family is big, and we've always been like this." In truth, you need to keep your focus on the growth and body mass index charts on pages xxxi to xxxiv. If your child's weight exceeds the normal range for his age and height, he meets the definition of being overweight or obese. It's not something that you can rationalize away.

There are certain metabolic or hormonal (endocrine) imbalances that often get blamed for weight problems. However, they are responsible for fewer than 1% of the cases of childhood obesity. Yes, hypothyroidism (a deficit in thyroid secretion) and other rarer and more severe genetic and metabolic disorders (eg, Prader-Willi syndrome, Turner syndrome, Cushing syndrome) can cause weight gain (and in some cases, other severe problems such as hearing and vision impairments). *You should certainly speak to your child's pediatrician about these concerns and a have a complete medical evaluation performed.* But because these syndromes are uncommon, they account for very few cases of obesity. More likely, your child's excess weight is associated with poor eating and activity habits, as well as certain parental and other issues that we'll discuss in this book.

"Because my child is heavy, he actually needs to eat more food to stay healthy." Based on this belief, many families may give bigger portions to the heavier children because of their size. Nothing could be more counterproductive. You need to rely on the growth charts and your pediatrician's advice and make sure that your child is consuming portion sizes that allow him to maintain an average weight. The sensible nutritional principles described in Chapter 2 should help keep your child's weight just where it should be.

Assessing Your Child's Obesity

Let's continue with the evaluation process that we began in the Introduction. This time, we'll consider where your youngster stands on a number of key contributors to childhood obesity. Take the answers to all of these questions with you on your next visit to the pediatrician's office and discuss them as you determine the best way to help your child reach and maintain an average weight.

Then, beginning with Chapter 2, we'll start to address your child's weight problem with specific strategies and approaches. We'll start with a discussion of good nutrition and how you can ensure that he eats well-balanced meals that can contribute to normal weight. You'll find some specific recommendations on issues like meal planning, food groups, and portion sizes that can help keep your child traveling along the right path to good health.

WORKSHEET TO TAKE TO YOUR PEDIATRICIAN

#5: YOUR CHILD'S GENETICS AND FAMILY HISTORY

How Does Family History Currently Influence Your Child's Health?
Let's look more closely at your own family. In the tables that follow, place a check mark beside the conditions and diseases of each family member. The more check marks you make, the greater your child's risk is of not only becoming overweight, but also of developing the serious diseases associated with it.

	Mother	Father	Sibling #1	Sibling #2	Sibling #3
Obese/overweight	☐	☐	☐	☐	☐
High blood pressure	☐	☐	☐	☐	☐
High cholesterol	☐	☐	☐	☐	☐
High triglycerides	☐	☐	☐	☐	☐
Diabetes	☐	☐	☐	☐	☐
Heart disease	☐	☐	☐	☐	☐
Asthma	☐	☐	☐	☐	☐
Joint pain	☐	☐	☐	☐	☐
Sleep apnea	☐	☐	☐	☐	☐
Liver disease	☐	☐	☐	☐	☐
Other _____	☐	☐	☐	☐	☐

Next, fill out a similar chart for your child's grandparents. Which of the following conditions apply to your youngster's grandfathers and grandmothers?

	Maternal Grandmother	Maternal Grandfather	Paternal Grandmother	Paternal Grandfather
Obese/overweight	☐	☐	☐	☐
High blood pressure	☐	☐	☐	☐
High cholesterol	☐	☐	☐	☐
High triglycerides	☐	☐	☐	☐
Diabetes	☐	☐	☐	☐
Heart disease	☐	☐	☐	☐
Asthma	☐	☐	☐	☐
Sleep apnea	☐	☐	☐	☐
Liver disease	☐	☐	☐	☐
Joint pain	☐	☐	☐	☐
Other _____	☐	☐	☐	☐

WORKSHEET TO TAKE TO YOUR PEDIATRICIAN
#6: ENVIRONMENTAL FACTORS

The following assessment will help you understand the environmental influences associated with your child's weight problem.

What Problems Exist Today (Home, School)?
Are there problems in your child's school/child care environment? _____

Are snacks healthy and portions controlled? _____

Is there time for outdoor play/recess? _____

Is there regular physical education at school? _____

Is there more than 1 to 2 hours of screen time (TV, computer)? _____

The Community Environment
Are there safe playgrounds and places to play outside in the neighborhood? _____

Are there after-school programs nearby that provide activity alternatives? _____

Are there opportunities to play sports/games at community centers? _____

Is it safe for your child to walk to school, activities, and friends' houses? _____

The Home Environment
Does the family have regularly scheduled TV/computer time? _____

Do family members regularly engage in physical activity together? _____

Is there an indoor and outdoor play space for the children? _____

Are there indoor activities your child can do at home instead of watching TV or using the computer? _____

Family Behavior
With family members in mind (including you, your spouse, and your child's siblings and grandparents), which of them

Overeats regularly _____

_____

Binges on food _____

_____

Rushes through meals _____

_____

Insists on keeping high-calorie snacks in the house _____

_____

Eats while watching TV _____

_____

Eats frequently at fast-food restaurants _____

_____

Overeats to calm anxiety _____

_____

Gets little or no physical activity each day _____

_____

Your Child's Behavior

Does your overweight child demonstrate the following behaviors that can contribute to an obesity problem? (Answer yes or no.)

Overeats regularly _____

Binges on food _____

Rushes through meals _____

Chooses high-calorie snacks _____

Selects high-sugar drinks _____

Eats while watching TV _____

Eats frequently at fast-food restaurants _____

Overeats to calm anxiety _____

Gets little or no physical activity each day _____

Sneaks or hides food _____

Seems hungry all the time _____

Gets upset when you try to limit portions or snacks _____

Watches more than 1 hour of TV/computer per day _____

Gets own food or snacks _____

Eats alone _____

Drinks a lot of sweetened beverages _____

2

What's to Eat?
The Importance of Good Nutrition

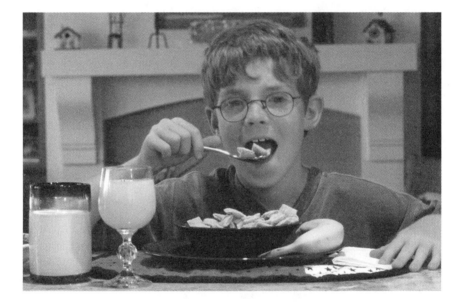

*W*hen parents think of the most important strategy for managing their children's weight, their attention often turns to the food they put on their children's plate and perhaps a formal diet or two that they've read about. This book takes a different approach than you might expect. Yes, your child's food consumption is a key factor in attaining a healthy weight. As you'll read, however, we're much more interested in good nutrition than in calorie counting or food restrictions.

The specific nutritional choices you and your youngster make are crucial, no matter her weight. Good nutrition is essential to good health and the American Academy of Pediatrics encourages parents to think of their nutritional decisions as *health* decisions. The nutritional choices for your child today will help determine her health not only now, but for the future. If you make an effort to feed her primarily healthy meals and snacks, you have a much better chance of helping her attain a healthy weight. Remember, your child's pediatrician will help you determine what a healthy weight is for your child, taking into account her age and height.

In short, if your child's weight has gotten ahead of her height, you shouldn't be putting a bandage on her weight problem. Instead, you need to be encouraging healthy eating habits that can last a lifetime. That means staying away from fad diets, including those in which deprivation is front and center. *Never* put your child's health at risk in exchange for weight loss.

Supporting Your Child's Growth

As you'll read in this chapter, all youngsters need a variety of foods high in nutritional value—from fruits and vegetables to whole grains and meat or fish—and a sufficient number of calories to grow properly. Infants and adolescents experience the most dramatic surges of childhood growth, but from the moment of birth, *all* children are always growing. In middle childhood, for example, there is a normal weight gain, averaging a little more than 6 pounds a year, that is accompanied by an annual increase in height of slightly more than 2 inches in boys and girls. Later, as puberty approaches, many children experience normal weight gains of 9 to 10 pounds annually. During these kinds of growth spurts, youngsters require more total calories and nutrients than usual. For this reason, even if your pediatrician has indicated that weight loss is an appropriate goal, you should *never* place your child on a calorie-restricted diet unless your pediatrician supervises it because strict caloric constraints can keep your youngster from consuming essential nutrients that she needs to grow. Keep in mind that calories are really just a measurement of the energy delivered by food, and your youngster requires energy to fuel her growth and power her physical activity.

At the same time, however, in the midst of the obesity epidemic that you read about in the Introduction, your pediatrician will encourage you to work toward an *energy* balance in your child's life—that is, balancing her daily calorie consumption with the amount of energy she expends. Too many parents create a nutritional environment at home filled with plenty of high-calorie snacks in the cupboards and lots of sugar-rich beverages in the refrigerator. They depend on their children to make the most appropriate choices from the array of tempting foods accessible to them. As a parent, you need to take a different approach. Just like you make an effort to child-proof your home (putting knifes and other sharp utensils in a latched drawer, keeping matches out of reach and out of sight), you need to create a healthy nutritional environment in which the burden isn't on your child to filter out the bad choices from the good ones. With only occasional exceptions, her food options should be limited to those that can contribute to overall healthy eating and energy balance.

In this chapter, you'll find guidelines that will help you put your child on a nutritional path that will serve her well. By familiarizing

Where the American Academy of Pediatrics Stands

The American Academy of Pediatrics feels strongly that healthy eating habits should begin in infancy and continue throughout childhood, adolescence, and beyond. As a parent, you have an enormous influence on your child's eating behaviors that can last a lifetime and can prevent or reduce the risk of obesity. Without your attention focused on what (and how much) she's eating, your child can begin to move in the direction of obesity in the first years of life.

If you are trying to help your obese child lose weight, *it is very important to do so under the supervision of your pediatrician.* Your pediatrician can monitor your child's progress and help ensure that she is maintaining an optimal energy balance in a healthy and safe manner. Your pediatrician can help guide you toward feeding your overweight child a balanced diet that along with regular physical activity, can produce a steady reduction in weight of about 1 pound a week.

yourself with ways to optimize her nutrition and creating a health-promoting eating plan for your entire family, you can ensure that your child isn't overfed and is eating the right kinds of foods in the right amounts to help her grow.

Organizing the Nutritional Environment

Weight loss won't happen on its own. To make sure your child is eating in an optimal way, you need to adopt a structured approach to her eating. That means doing some planning for the food that she eats—breakfast, lunch, dinner, and snacks. It may mean using MyPyramid (formerly known as the Food Guide Pyramid) and other information in this chapter to thoughtfully prepare meals that are balanced and have portion sizes appropriate for your child's age. Remember, as her parent, you're in charge of the nutritional environment at home. You should decide the foods that come into your home and what will be served and when. When you prepare age-appropriate portions of a nutritionally balanced diet for your child at meals and snacks, she can learn to listen to her own hunger signals and choose how much to eat, and you will know that she has the appropriate balance and amount of food needed for her growth and development. This is an opportunity to set a good example, such as providing at least one fruit or vegetable with every meal. With an older child, begin to involve her by discussing what she would choose for healthy meals and snacks. As children grow into teenagers, they have more opportunities to make decisions about what they will eat. Encouraging them and praising them for making healthy food choices is a good way to help them make this transition.

In some ways, this approach to weight loss is probably different than what you've been used to in the past. When the goal is lowering the number on the bathroom scale, most people are accustomed to counting calories. But as we've already noted, caloric restriction can be potentially risky in growing children. Thus, our emphasis here will always be on good nutrition and avoiding low-value foods such as high-calorie snacks and high-sugar drinks, not on consciously limiting calories.

Food Groups and MyPyramid

As an adult, you've probably heard about the major food groups many times, although you might not have used them in meal planning—until now. The good news is that all 5 of the major food groups have many healthy choices for your child (see below). It's important to include a variety of foods from the food groups in your youngster's diet.

Choices From the Major Food Groups

Here are examples of foods from the 5 major food groups.

- *Grains:* whole-grain breads, oatmeal, brown rice, pasta, potatoes
- *Dairy products:* skim or low-fat (1%) milk, low-fat yogurt, reduced-fat cheese, cottage cheese
- *Vegetables:* beets, broccoli, carrots, green beans, peas, spinach, vegetable juices
- *Fruits:* bananas, apples, pears, strawberries, cantaloupes, raisins, watermelons, fruit juice
- *Meat/protein:* lean cuts of beef, skinless poultry, fish, eggs, peanut butter, beans, reduced-fat deli meats, tofu

Every food group is important to providing essential nutrients and energy that can support normal growth, good health, and sensible weight management.

One way to help ensure that your child is eating from all the major food groups is to refer to the online MyPyramid as you're planning and preparing meals. Created by the US Department of Agriculture, MyPyramid is based on the government's dietary recommendations *(Dietary Guidelines for Americans),* which were updated most recently in 2005. MyPyramid is designed for the general population—specifically, for healthy people older than 2 years—and depicts food selections from each of the food groups and the minimum number of servings your child should eat from each group.

The newest version of MyPyramid provides recommendations on the number, type, and size of food servings. For personalized information, you'll need to access the interactive system on the government's Web site, www.mypyramid.gov. In one of the Web site's features, you can insert your child's age, gender, and activity level and be given specific dietary guidelines. For example, a 7-year-old girl who is physically active for 30 to 60 minutes on most days should aim for 5 ounces of grains, 2 cups of vegetables, 1.5 cups of fruits, 3 cups of milk, and 5 ounces of meat and beans per day. A 14-year-old boy who exercises less than 30 minutes on most days should consume 6 ounces of grains, 2.5 cups of vegetables, 2 cups of fruits, 3 cups of milk, and 5.5 ounces of meat and beans per day.

If you use MyPyramid as a road map to what your child should eat, she'll get all the nutrients she needs. Keep in mind, however, that MyPyramid is a *guide,* not a prescription—your child doesn't necessarily have to eat the precise number of servings on MyPyramid *every day*. However, over the course of 1 to 2 weeks, her daily intake should average the number of recommended servings. Again, the goal is to keep your child moving along the proper path of consuming healthy foods and well-balanced meals; the calories and her weight loss will take care of themselves, particularly if your child is physically active each day.

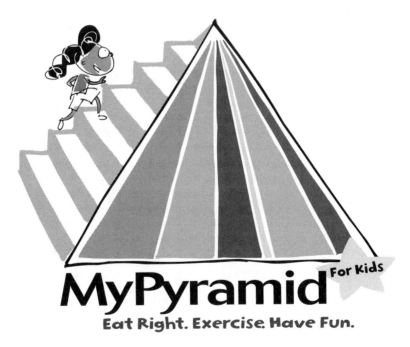

Source: United States Department of Agriculture, 2005

Components of Your Child's Diet

No matter what your child's weight is, most of her daily calories (about 55%–60% of them) should come from carbohydrates, primarily complex carbohydrates. In fact, the main dishes at mealtime should stress these complex carbohydrates.

As for dietary fats, the new US Department of Agriculture guidelines recommend that young children (2–3 years old) should have a fat intake comprising 30% to 35% of their total calories, while older children and adolescents (4–18 years old) should have between 25% and 35% of their calories come from fats.

Here is a brief description of the major food categories.

- *Carbohydrates* are the major fuel for physical performance. The new dietary guidelines (www.mypyramid.gov) recommend that half the intake of grain come from whole grains (complex carbohydrates), including whole wheat bread, brown rice, wild rice, and whole wheat pasta. When you look at a food label, the words "whole" or "whole grain" will come before the name of the grain.
- *Protein* is the major building block of the body, necessary for growth and repair of human tissue. Protein is found in foods such as milk, cheese, meat, and beans.
- *Fat* is needed by the body in modest amounts throughout the lifespan—but before a child is 2 years old, it should not be restricted. Fat is a vital component of cell membranes and supports the absorption of the fat-soluble vitamins A, D, E, and K. Meat and dairy products contain fat, as do vegetable oils, fish oil, and peanut butter.

Portion and Serving Sizes

We live in a culture in which many restaurants are renowned for supersizing virtually every item on their menu and parents often overestimate the amount of food that their children need. That kind of thinking can put youngsters on the fast track to obesity.

Keep in mind that your child does not require the same serving size as an adult. In the same way, portion sizes should be different for a 5-year-old and a 15-year-old. Even so, many parents remain confused over how big their children's servings should be. The key here is to feed age-appropriate portions to your youngster. As a general guideline, the Table on page 28 suggests age-appropriate portion and serving sizes across the various food groups.

Dietary Guidelines for Americans 2005 provides some guidance, issuing some of its recommendations in specific serving sizes rather than as number of servings. Additional information for your own child can be found on www.mypyramid.gov.

For more specifics, ask your pediatrician. In fact, you should not make any drastic changes in the amount your child eats until you discuss it with your pediatrician.

Feeding Guide for Children*

Food	Age, y 2 to 3 Portion Size	2 to 3 Servings	4 to 6 Portion Size	4 to 6 Servings	7 to 12 Portion Size	7 to 12 Servings	Comments
Milk and dairy	1/2 c (4 oz)	4–5 16–20 oz total	1/2–3/4 c (4–6 oz)	3–4 24–32 oz total	1/2–1 c (4–8 oz)	3–4 24–32 oz total	The following may be substituted for 1/2 c fluid milk: 1/2–3/4 oz cheese, 1/2 cup yogurt, 2 1/2 tbsp nonfat dry milk
Meat, fish, poultry, or equivalent	1–2 oz	2 2–4 oz total	1–2 oz	2 2–4 oz total	2 oz	3–4 6–8 oz total	The following may be substituted for 1 oz meat, fish, or poultry: 1 egg, 2 tbsp peanut butter, 4–5 tbsp cooked legumes
Vegetables and fruit		4–5		4–5		3–4	Include one green leafy or yellow vegetable for vitamin A, such as carrots, spinach, broccoli, winter squash, or greens
Vegetables Cooked	2–3 tbsp		3–4 tbsp		1/4–1/2 c		
Raw†	Few pieces		Few Pieces		Several pieces		
Fruit Raw	1/2–1 small		1/2–1 small		1 medium		Include one vitamin C-rich fruit, vegetable, or juice, such as citrus juices, orange, grapefruit, strawberries, melon, tomato, or broccoli
Canned	2–4 tbsp		4–6 tbsp		1/4–1/2 c		
Juice	3–4 oz		4 oz		4 oz		
Grain products Whole grain or enriched bread	1/2–1 slice	3–4	1 slice	3–4	1 slice	4–5	The following may be substituted for 1 slice of bread: 1/2 c spaghetti, macaroni, noodles, or rice; 5 saltines; 1/2 English muffin or bagel; 1 tortilla; corn grits or posole
Cooked cereal	1/4–1/2 c		1/2 c		1/2–1 c		
Dry cereal	1/2–1 c		1 c		1 c		

*Adapted from Lowenberg ME. Development of food patterns in young children. In: Pipes PL, Trahms CM, eds. *Nutrition Infancy and Childhood.* 5th ed. St Louis, MO: Mosby-Year Book; 1993:168–169. With permission of Elsevier.
†Do not give to young children until they can chew well.

Portion Sizes

These illustrations depict the 5 major food groups on the plates of children of various ages. They will give you some perspective on the portion sizes that may be appropriate for your own child.

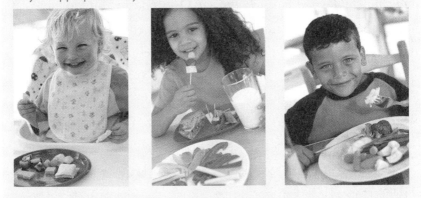

One way to help avoid serving excessively large portion sizes to your child is to make sure that there are a variety of food groups on her plate. If you serve her a protein source such as chicken, 2 vegetables, and pasta for dinner, there simply won't be room on her plate to overdo it on the pasta, for example.

You should also encourage your child to eat slowly. Some overweight children race through their meals and have no idea how much they're really eating. By slowing down the pace, an older child in particular will be able to judge whether she is still hungry. She'll be giving her brain the chance to recognize that she has eaten enough to feel satisfied, and when she's no longer hungry, she's more likely to stop eating. Also, by taking smaller bites and chewing her food more thoroughly, she'll enjoy her food more.

By eating together as a family, you can help your child with healthy eating habits as well as provide valuable family together time. Keep meals pleasant and focus on the positives. *Remember that your job is to provide nutritional, well-balanced meals in the proper portions, and your child will decide what to eat.* Overfocusing on food and eating can be replaced by finding out what happened at school and with their friends and leave time for family interactions.

Nutritional Balance

Nutritional balance is the key. All food groups contain essential nutrients for your child's growth and health. The key to a healthy weight is choosing the appropriate amounts of each food. Focusing on only one food group as the culprit can lead to an imbalance in meeting nutritional needs. That's not to say that you don't have to watch out for excess snack foods, sugared beverages, and large portions, but try to offer a balanced approach and limit high-calorie sweets and treats by only having these foods in small amounts for special occasions. Rely more often on foods like

- Fresh fruits and vegetables
- Whole grain breads and cereals
- Low-fat and nonfat dairy products (eg, milk and yogurt)
- Moderate portions of skim-milk cheeses
- Lean meats (eg, chicken, turkey, lean beef cuts, lean pork cuts)
- Fish
- Pretzels, baked tortilla chips, and baked potato chips
- Frozen fruit bars and angel food cake instead of rich, creamy desserts

Making Smart Shopping Choices

If you're like most parents, you probably don't have time to do as much menu planning as you'd like. Thus, you may feel that the decisions you make in the supermarket occur in the spur of the moment much too often. Keep in mind, however, that most supermarkets carry thousands of food items on their shelves, and impulse buying can be risky. You may end up purchasing foods that you really had no intention of buying.

For that reason, it pays to have a plan. Find a few minutes before you shop to make a list of the basic items you need, concentrating on the healthy foods described in this chapter. It's also a good idea to shop at a market that you're familiar with, where you know the location of most of the foods you want. You'll spend less time browsing down the aisles, where you may find and choose foods that your family really doesn't need.

When you enter the market, concentrate first on shopping along its outer borders, where most stores keep fresh fruits and vegetables, dairy products, meats, and juices. Packaged items, which are often higher in calories, tend to be on interior shelves. Invite your older child to shop with you to learn about nutrition labels and be an active participant in selecting healthy foods. Just prior to purchasing your groceries, spend a moment that might be called "Right Before Checkout," looking into your cart and making sure that you actually want all the items that are there.

By the way, optimal food selection is only the first step in this process. Once you're in the kitchen and preparing meals, be sure to trim all visible fat from meat and remove the skin from chicken before cooking. Also, use cooking techniques such as broiling, roasting, and steaming that call for little or no fat. If your family likes butter or margarine on cooked vegetables, try to add only small amounts or use healthy oils such as seasoning with a bit of olive oil or pesto sauce.

Eating on the Run

You know the feeling—you're rushing in the morning to get your children off to school, you're hurrying in the afternoon to drive them to soccer practice, and you're racing home from work in the evening to make sure they have time for a study session at a friend's house.

When something's got to give in a schedule like that, it's often family meals. Many families never sit down at the dining room table even once during the day. When everyone is eating on the run or the kids are having some of their meals or snacks away from home (eg, at a child care center, at friends' homes), that's when healthy foods can give way to the easier, higher fat, higher calorie choices. Sound familiar?

Even if there never seem to be enough hours in the day for your family to eat as healthfully as you'd like, don't despair. Here are some suggestions to help keep your overweight child on the right track.

- Plan ahead for those times when you know you're going to be busy. If it means spending time on the weekend preparing meals for the upcoming weekdays, then do it.
- Sit together at the table for meals as a family whenever possible to eat and talk together.
- Discuss how the family can decrease eating out at fast-food restaurants.

- Fix breakfast the night before. You can precook hard-boiled eggs or have your child's favorite cold cereal already in the bowl and the fresh fruit sliced and ready to go at the crack of dawn.

- Keep things simple. You don't have to cook an elaborate dinner every night. For example, why not prepare a bowl of soup, a sandwich, and a salad, topping the meal off with a piece of fruit and a glass of nonfat milk, on evenings when you're particularly rushed? It will provide your child with a nutritious meal without pushing yourself to the point of collapse. The key is to make good nutritional choices, no matter how simple or extravagant the meal is.

- When your child spends time at friends' homes, why not call the parents of your youngster's friends and offer to send over healthy foods or snacks for all the kids? Turkey sandwiches or apples may keep your child from grabbing higher fat choices that her friends might otherwise offer.

- For a youngster who goes to a child care center or after-school program or eats at the school cafeteria, you need to find out what the nutritional environment is like there. If the menu relies too often on cheeseburgers and french fries, your child needs to bring her own meals and snacks from home. At the same time, talk to your school or child care administrator about improving the nutritional choices. Don't forget about the school vending machines, either; if they're weighed down with candy and soft drinks, you and other parents should lobby for an improvement in the available selections.

The Perils of Fast Food

Fast-food restaurants have permeated every corner of the United States and are probably in the consciousness of nearly every US child. Many TV ads for these eating establishments are targeted specifically at children, and so are the promotional toys and the playgrounds that are part of the restaurant offerings. As a result, millions of kids persuade their parents to line up their cars at the drive-through window several days a week—and in a fast-paced world in which adults and children alike often seem to have too much squeezed into their days, parents are only too happy to give in to the convenience of the local fast-food restaurant from time to time. In fact, 1 of every 10 food dollars is currently spent at fast-food establishments, adding up to a collective food bill of more than $34 billion annually. In many families, 40% of the family food budget is spent eating outside of the home.

Yes, it's possible to make nutritious fast-food selections. But let's face it—there are many more high-fat, high-sugar, high-calorie choices, from hamburgers to fries to shakes, often served in king-size portions that can sabotage your child's best efforts to control her weight. Fast foods often don't supply a healthy balance of vitamins and minerals and are frequently very high in salt.

When you do take the kids to a fast-food restaurant, talk with them in advance about making healthier choices. Fast food doesn't necessarily have to be bad food; good selections may include

- A grilled or charbroiled chicken sandwich (without the skin and mayonnaise)
- A regular-sized hamburger (not the large one with all the fixings)

- A salad with a small amount of salad dressing
- A plain baked potato (perhaps topped with vegetables from the salad bar)
- Skim or 1% (low-fat) milk or orange juice (rather than a high-fat shake or soda)

If your child must have fries, divide a single order among several members of the family. (Some chains now cook their french fries in vegetable oil rather than animal fat.)

Your child may love fast-food fare, and it can seem like the breather you need at the end of an exhausting day. But if you do the math, you might be surprised that fast-food dining is actually pretty expensive. If it costs $20 or $25 to feed a family of 4 at a fast-food restaurant, and if you eat there 3 or 4 times a week, that can take a supersized bite out of the family budget. You need to ask yourself whether you could take that same money and buy more nutritious food for your family. On those days when the family does eat out, avoid fast food and consider splitting portions, which are often too large. It is wise to steer clear of buffets that can tempt everyone to eating too large of portions and second helpings.

One other important suggestion—eat as many of your meals at home as possible. When you or another adult in the home does the cooking, there is more control over what your child eats. Turn those trips to the fast-food restaurant into a once-in-a-while treat, not an everyday outing. When you have the opportunity to sit down for a meal as a family, grab it.

The Power of Incremental Changes

A lot of diet programs ask people to transform the way they eat and make these major changes overnight. Not surprisingly, most individuals have trouble sticking to those kinds of dramatic shifts in their diets, particularly over the long term. Eating habits develop over many years, and they can be hard to change.

For that reason, our recommendations here are quite different. When it comes to your overweight child, you need to help her make *gradual, small* changes in her eating habits over a period of time. Introduce 1 or 2 changes a week. She'll find those kinds of changes— a little at a time—are the easiest kinds to make.

We've already given you some ideas to help make this transition in slow and steady increments. For example, it could mean eating out at restaurants less often—perhaps twice a week rather than 4 or 5 times a week. Or you might order a small hamburger or grilled chicken sandwich for your child rather than the titanic-sized burger. Here are some other suggestions for incremental dietary changes.

- Introduce new, healthier foods over a period of time. Some children are resistant to try any new food; it may take multiple attempts before they develop a taste for it.
- Evaluate what snack foods your family is eating, and gradually move them in the direction of healthier alternatives—for example, unsalted pretzels rather than potato chips, air-popped popcorn instead of cookies, and frozen juice bars (without added sugar) instead of ice cream.
- Serve salads more often, and choose low-fat salad dressing. Teach children about an appropriate amount of salad dressing to use and how they can order it on the side at restaurants.

- When making sandwiches, use low-fat meats (eg, turkey ham, turkey) and see if your child notices the difference.
- Switch from mayonnaise and other high-fat spreads to reduced-fat varieties. Use spreads sparingly and teach your child to do the same.
- Try out a child-friendly vegetarian recipe for spaghetti or lasagna, using vegetables instead of meat, along with lower fat cheeses.
- Gradually substitute water or low-calorie beverages for higher calorie drinks.

All in the Family

As we'll emphasize throughout this book, helping your child lose weight should be a family project. You can't expect your obese youngster to change her eating habits on her own while others in the household are showing no self-restraint and continuing to reach for candy and high-fat ice cream. Children are just too smart to accept a "Do as I say, not as I do" attitude from their parents and other family members.

So your *entire* family needs to get on board supporting the weight-loss efforts of your obese youngster. That means modeling healthy eating behaviors that you want your child to adopt, now and in the future. It means recruiting all the adults in your child's life as well as your other children as active members of the support team who are setting a good example, day by day. Everyone should be adopting the same eating plan, or you'll risk making your overweight child feel singled out, isolated, and even resentful and increase the chances of failure.

Now, what if you have an overweight youngster in your family, but your other children are not? How do you explain to a thin child that the entire family is adopting a new way of eating, even if she has no need to lose weight herself? Here is the approach that we recommend. Explain that the entire family is going to work at getting *healthier* and that the nutritional changes being made are for the well-being of the *entire* family, from the thinnest to the most overweight ("We're going to have strawberries for dessert tonight instead of chocolate cake because it's a lot healthier for *all* of us.").

At the same time, turn mealtime into family time whenever possible. Try eating most of your meals together. Children learn more about good food choices and healthy nutrition when family members join one another for breakfast, lunch, and dinner. Research also shows that kids eat more vegetables and fruits and consume fewer fried foods and sugary drinks when they eat with the entire family.

As you use the recommendations in this chapter to change the way your child eats, she'll find that this new nutritional approach becomes easier with time. Remember, you don't need to count calories or fat grams, and you don't need to panic if your child has a bad day or even a bad week. A little backsliding isn't going to derail a good eating plan if she gets back on track as soon as possible. Remember that energy balance is the long-term goal.

Choosing Healthy Snacks

If the snacks at your home have usually been cookies, doughnuts, and soft drinks, it's time for a change. Two or 3 snacks a day are an important part of your child's overall nutrition, so you need to make them just as nutritionally sound as her regular meals, while contributing to an overall program aimed at weight loss. Planning snacks ahead of time is helpful—prepackage some appropriate servings to have ready for kids in their lunches or when they get home from school. This is an opportunity to teach healthy choices and practices.

If you keep the pantry, refrigerator, and kitchen table stocked with plenty of low-fat, low-sugar snacks from the 5 major food groups, that's what she'll reach for. Of course, occasional treats like ice cream are fine. But for those snacks that your child typically grabs on her own, make sure they're nutritious ones such as

- Fruit
- Low-fat/frozen yogurt
- Celery stalks
- Low-fat oatmeal cookies
- Cucumber slices
- Frozen bananas
- Baked potato chips
- Bran muffins
- Fresh strawberries
- Air-popped popcorn
- Low-fat cheeses
- Frozen juice bars (without added sugar)
- Crackers
- Sugar-free cereals
- Unsalted pretzels
- Dried raisins or apricots

Adding a protein food with these snacks can make them more satisfying. Try adding a boiled egg, cheese stick, yogurt, natural peanut butter, or nuts (if your child is old enough so choking is not a concern).

WORKSHEET TO TAKE TO YOUR PEDIATRICIAN

#7: HOW IS YOUR CHILD EATING NOW?

To help produce lasting improvements in a child's weight, many parents find it helpful to keep a food diary to monitor exactly what the child is eating. Toward that end, use this worksheet for the next 4 days to record what your child eats, from the time he or she awakens to when he or she goes to sleep.

Foods Eaten Today (enter date): _____

Under each meal and snack write down *what* and *how much* your child ate.

Breakfast _____

Mid-morning Snack _____

Lunch _____

Afternoon Snack _____

Juice or Soda _____

Dinner _____

Late-night Snack _____

Foods Eaten Today (enter date): _____

Under each meal and snack write down *what* and *how much* your child ate.

Breakfast _____

Mid-morning Snack _____

Lunch _____

Afternoon Snack _____

Juice or Soda _____

Dinner _____

Late-night Snack _____

Foods Eaten Today (enter date): _____

Under each meal and snack write down *what* and *how much* your child ate.

Breakfast _____

Mid-morning Snack _____

Lunch _____

Afternoon Snack _____

Juice or Soda _____

Dinner _____

Late-night Snack _____

Foods Eaten Today (enter date): _____

Under each meal and snack write down *what* and *how much* your child ate.

Breakfast _____

Mid-morning Snack _____

Lunch _____

Afternoon Snack _____

Juice or Soda _____

Dinner _____

Late-night Snack _____

WORKSHEET TO TAKE TO YOUR PEDIATRICIAN
#8: WHAT NUTRITIONAL PROBLEMS EXIST?

Once you become increasingly familiar with the path toward healthier eating, review the food diaries (worksheet #7) to determine how your child is faring.

Are improvements needed in areas such as
- ☐ Eating plenty of whole grains
- ☐ Consuming low-fat dairy products
- ☐ Eating 5 fruits and vegetables daily
- ☐ Avoiding sugary drinks
- ☐ Staying away from high-fat snacks
- ☐ Reducing visits to fast-food restaurants
- ☐ Keeping portion sizes at age-appropriate levels

What Changes Need to Be Made?
It's time to climb on the fast track toward improving your child's diet. Use the information in Chapter 2 to help you identify changes that you and your child can make to move in the direction of healthier eating.

To get started, alter your diet a step at a time. If you try to do too much too soon, you might get stuck in one area or another, and become discouraged with all of your efforts. Use the following space to define a single dietary area you'd like to change and your strategy for doing so. Once you've been successful, move on to another nutritional area that needs changing.

What one area of the family's diet do I want to change first? (For example, you may want to decrease the family's intake of sugar-sweetened juice or soft drinks.)

_____

_____

How do I plan to do this? (Be specific. For example, if you want to reduce juice and soft drinks, you may need to plan on sending water to school for your child's snack instead of juice and having water or noncaloric beverages available at home instead of juice or soda.)

_____

_____

As you and your child begin to make these changes, who can join you on this journey and offer support in these efforts?

_____

_____

Once you have one change under your belt, decide on the next change, how you will accomplish this change, and who can help.

_____

_____

In the days and weeks ahead, continue to use food diaries (worksheet #7) to monitor how your child is doing. Write down what your youngster is eating during meals and snacks as soon as possible after that food is consumed, and use this information to keep track of your child's progress and the changes he or she has been able to make.

What Is Going Well?
On a regular basis, evaluate the improvements your child is making on the journey toward better health. Every week or two, ask yourself questions like

Have you seen changes and improvements in your child's eating? _____

In what ways is your child eating more healthfully? _____

How many food group servings does your child consume during a typical day?

Whole grains _____   Fruits _____

Dairy products _____   Meat/protein _____

Vegetables _____

Are there additional dietary changes you plan to make in the days and weeks ahead?

_____

_____

Throughout this book, we'll refer back to the information on these worksheets to determine whether you and your child have made changes that can move your child in the direction of healthier food choices.

WORKSHEET TO TAKE TO YOUR PEDIATRICIAN
#9: IS YOUR CHILD EATING MORE HEALTHFULLY?

Now that you're becoming familiar with the path to healthier eating, use the food diaries on this worksheet to record the progress your child is making in the way he or she eats. As you did with the food diaries on worksheet #7, write down *what* and *how much* your youngster is eating during meals and snacks as soon as possible after that food is consumed.

Foods Eaten Today (enter date): _____

Breakfast _____

Mid-morning Snack _____

Lunch _____

Afternoon Snack _____

Juice or Soda _____

Dinner _____

Late-night Snack _____

How many food group servings has your child consumed during the day?

Whole grains _____   Fruits _____

Dairy products _____   Meat/protein _____

Vegetables _____

Foods Eaten Today (enter date): _____

Breakfast _____

Mid-morning Snack _____

Lunch _____

Afternoon Snack _____

Juice or Soda _____

Dinner _____

Late-night Snack _____

How many food group servings has your child consumed during the day?

Whole grains _____   Fruits _____

Dairy products _____   Meat/protein _____

Vegetables _____

Foods Eaten Today (enter date): _____

Breakfast _____

Mid-morning Snack _____

Lunch _____

Afternoon Snack _____

Juice or Soda _____

Dinner _____

Late-night Snack _____

How many food group servings has your child consumed during the day?

Whole grains _____   Fruits _____

Dairy products _____   Meat/protein _____

Vegetables _____

(Worksheet continued on page 46)

Now compare the entries in these new food diaries with those that you filled out earlier (worksheet #7).

Have you seen changes and an improvement in your child's eating? _____

In what ways is your child eating more healthfully?

_____

_____

What other dietary changes do you plan to make in the days and weeks ahead?

_____

_____

3

Physical Activity: Ready, Set, Be Fit!

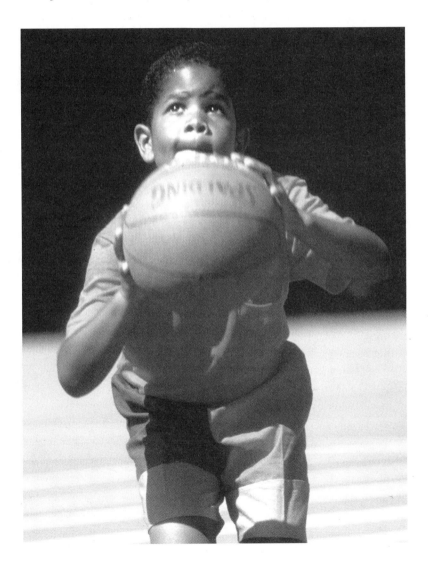

A generation ago, most parents didn't give much thought to whether their children were physically active. In many of those families, the kids came home from school, had a snack, and then headed outdoors to play with friends until they were called in for dinner. Most children, it seemed, were constantly active without much or any coaxing.

Times have changed. Today, millions of US children are driven to school and just about everywhere else they need to go. At school, they may spend more time sitting and less time moving, thanks to cutbacks in physical education (PE) classes. At home, their parents may not give them household chores that could keep them active. And they've traded in afternoons at the playground for hours spent playing video games or watching TV.

Unfortunately, children are paying the price for all that time spent operating the remote control and computer joystick. As you've already read, there's an epidemic of obesity, and the waning interest in physical activity is a big reason why. After all, with children spending an average of 3 hours a day in front of the TV or computer screen, they're not playing, running, jumping, or otherwise being physically active. Television watching is a completely sedentary activity (or inactivity, to be more accurate). To make matters worse, many children snack while they're sitting in front of the television. No wonder every hour a child spends on the couch is an hour that can contribute to his obesity problem. That's why the American Academy of Pediatrics (AAP) urges you to help your overweight child understand the importance of physical activity and encourage him to choose to be active every day.

Physical Activity = Better Health

Pediatricians continue to be disturbed by the trends they're seeing in the levels of physical activity of children, which appear to be headed in the wrong direction. One survey concluded that less than 25% of children in grades 4 through 12 participate in 20 minutes of vigorous activity or 30 minutes of any physical activity per day. Particularly with weight management as a goal, those numbers aren't good enough.

Not only will regular physical activity help your child lose weight and maintain that weight loss, but it has many other benefits. For example, if your child exercises regularly, he'll have

- Stronger bones and joints
- Greater muscle strength
- A decrease in body fat
- Improved flexibility
- A healthier cardiovascular system (thus reducing his risk of developing heart disease and high blood pressure)
- A reduced likelihood of developing diabetes
- More energy
- A greater ability to handle stress
- Improvements in self-confidence and self-esteem
- Greater social acceptance by physically active peers
- Opportunities to make new friends
- Better concentration at school

Getting Started

You should have a clear picture of your child's activity level—and whether he needs to change course. Is he watching too much TV? Is he spending too little time playing outdoors after school or on weekends?

As a parent, you need to help your overweight child get moving. To repeat, he should be doing some physical activity every day. In fact, it should become as routine a part of his life as brushing his teeth and sleeping.

So where should you begin? How much time does your child need to spend being active and how intense does this activity need to be?

The answers to these questions may be different for your child than it is for another boy or girl. If your overweight youngster has been completely sedentary, with no PE classes at school, no outdoor play, no extracurricular physical activities, and hours of TV watching every day, his starting point should be different than that of a fairly active youngster. There are plenty of activities that he can choose from, and he should begin to slowly and gradually pick up the pace.

Let's say that your child decides to try getting his physical activity by taking walks or hikes with an older sibling through a nearby park. If he is really out of shape or if he has trouble imagining doing any walking at all, encourage him to set a goal of walking for only 1 minute at a time ("Can you walk for just 60 seconds?"). Once he realizes that 1 minute is an attainable target, have him increase his walking sessions progressively, to 2 minutes each time, then

3 minutes, and so on, until he's walking for 30 minutes or more. If your youngster is already in better shape, he may want to start with a 15-minute walk and then increase it in 5-minute increments to 20 minutes, 25 minutes, and beyond. The ultimate goal is to have him spend an hour being active each day.

To most of us, a minute or two of walking doesn't sound like much. In fact, many adolescents and adults think that exercise doesn't really count unless it's intense and even hurts (as the cliché goes, "No pain, no gain"). But for a child trying to lose weight, every little bit of activity helps, whether it's a short walk to the school bus stop or a climb up a flight of stairs at school. Ultimately, once your child gets into better shape, you can encourage him to increase the duration and intensity of his activity, but the most important thing is that he just get moving and do it regularly.

What Activity Should Your Child Choose?

There are a lot of avenues for your overweight child to pursue in the quest to become more active. From Little League baseball to ballet lessons, shooting a basketball to bicycling, he has many options to choose from. And that's the key—*your child,* not you, should be the person making the choice. If he's going to stay active long term, he needs to select something that he likes and will keep doing.

That's why it's important for parents not to micromanage their children's physical activities. Some children enjoy organized activity, while others prefer outdoor free play for which they're left to their own devices on how they'll be active. Free play can be a powerful form of exercise, contributing to the development of motor skills and serving as a great outlet for your youngster's energy. As a society, we're overlooking the value of this kind of active play, even though the AAP recommends *only* free play, rather than team sports, up to the age of 6 years. Whether you live in a city or rural area, find a park, playground, or other outdoor area where your young child can do his own thing.

Yes, you can make sure that some balls and other play equipment are available whenever your child goes outside, but let him decide exactly what he wants to do. Parents often find it helpful to give their children 3 or 4 activity options from which to choose, or they might ask their youngsters what choices they'd like available.

Pose a question like this to your child: "If you weren't watching TV, what could you be doing instead?" Don't be surprised if you initially get a blank stare from him, so give him some concrete alternatives: "Could you jump rope? Or play tennis? Or go in-line skating? Or go for a brisk walk?"

You might instead say, "Here are 3 activities you could do this afternoon. You could swim, go bowling with your brother, or go for a walk. Which one would you like to do?"

On the other hand, if you *insist* that your child participate in an activity that he finds boring or grueling—"Jimmy, it's time to walk on the treadmill!"—he'll probably lose interest quickly and end up in front of the TV. If you provide him the opportunity to participate in an activity that he enjoys, he's likely to keep doing it.

Now, what about organized sports like soccer teams and Little League? They're fine for children aged 6 years and older who want to join in, but it's important to have realistic expectations. Your aim should be for your child to be physically active and enjoy the experience, not necessarily excel as the best player on the team. You shouldn't be trying to create an elite athlete, and if he chooses to move from one sport to another rather than concentrating only on one, that's fine. For example, if he shows an interest in a basketball league, great—but if he also wants to learn how to ski when winter comes around, all the better. Let him explore different activities. He'll develop a wide variety of physical skills and more importantly, he'll keep moving.

Here are some other guidelines to keep in mind when selecting activities with your child.

- Anything that involves movement qualifies as physical activity. It doesn't have to push your child to the point of collapse to contribute to his efforts at weight management.
- When you present your child with alternatives or options for activities, create the boundaries of acceptable choices. Perhaps joining the hockey team is too expensive for your family budget—not only the sign-up fee, but the cost of the skates and other equipment. There are plenty of other choices that should be within your family's financial means.
- While many youngsters love being active with other kids, some overweight children feel self-conscious or embarrassed about participating in group sports. They may be more inclined to choose an activity that they can do on their own. Another approach is to plan physical activities for your youngster together with a special friend or sibling with whom he feels comfortable.
- Above all, the activity must be fun, and your child should be successful at it.

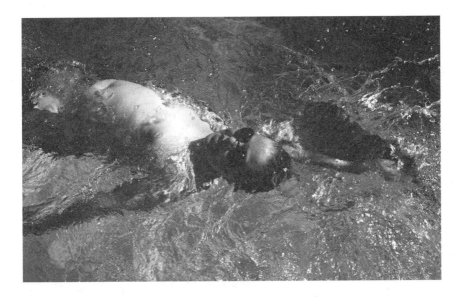

What's Right for Your Child?

There's no scarcity of activities that you can make available to your child, and *all* kids can find some form of exercise that they enjoy, even if they tell you that they'd much rather sit and snack on the couch. You'll find many of these options mentioned throughout this chapter. You can also use your imagination to add to the list of appropriate choices for your own child, perhaps including hiking, gardening, snorkeling, gymnastics, stair climbing, or playing with a hula hoop. You can get him a dog if he agrees to walk his new pet twice a day. You could also buy him a basketball and put up a hoop in your driveway. Remember, even household chores—from raking leaves to vacuuming the house to washing the car—qualify as physical activity as long as they keep your child moving.

(continued on page 56)

Don't overlook youth activities sponsored by your community's parks and recreation department, which might include volleyball, badminton, or table tennis. Encourage your youngster to stay active by giving him gifts like riding lessons. At his birthday parties, incorporate some physical activity, perhaps by taking his friends and him to play miniature golf or planning a trip to the batting cages to swing at baseballs.

Also, keep in mind that there are lifetime sports that he can develop a love for and continue doing throughout his lifetime. If you can get your child interested in an activity like this when he's young, exercise and fitness are more likely to become a habit that lasts for many decades. In fact, the American Academy of Pediatrics recommends that physical education programs in schools emphasize lifetime sports (as well as activities that are not just for the best athletes). These lifetime sports include

- Swimming
- Golf
- Bicycling
- Jogging

- Racquetball
- Bowling
- Tennis
- Walking

- In-line and ice skating
- Skiing
- Martial arts

No matter what activity your child chooses, whether it burns lots of body fat or just a little, it is better than just sitting. That's the message to communicate to a child who wants to lose weight.

The Activity Pyramid

To help your youngster choose physical activities that are right for him, you might try using the Activity Pyramid (see page 58). This pyramid is based on guidelines developed by the Centers for Disease Control and Prevention and the American College of Sports Medicine and has been adapted by many health organizations and universities. Like MyPyramid in Chapter 2, it is a visually appealing way to teach children the importance of a balanced diet of physical activity and ways to make activity part of their lives.

As you can see, the Activity Pyramid divides activities into 6 groups, each of which represents a particular level or type of movement or exercise. For example,

- The greatest amount of space in the pyramid, its base, is devoted to activities that should be done most frequently. These are unstructured, from playing outside to giving your pet a bath, and can be done daily.
- Moving up the pyramid, the next 2 levels include aerobic activities like bicycling and in-line skating that get the heart pumping continuously for an extended period of time and recreational activities like kickball and volleyball. The pyramid recommends engaging in these activities 3 to 5 times a week.
- Closer to the top of the pyramid, there are 2 levels with leisure or playtime activities (for example, tumbling, miniature golf) and strength and flexibility exercises (for example, dancing, martial arts), which can be done 2 to 3 times per week.
- Finally, the top level shows activities (or more specifically, inactivities) that children may become involved in, from TV watching to playing computer games; the key is to do these inactivities less often.

(continued on page 58)

Bear in mind that the pyramid represents goals that your child can work toward. When he is just starting to incorporate physical activity into his life, he won't be able to meet all the recommendations in the pyramid. But he can get started by selecting activities he enjoys from various levels of the pyramid.

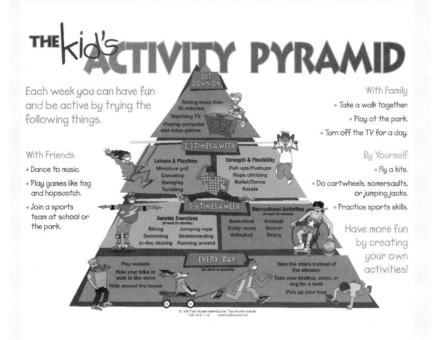

The Kid's Activity Pyramid © 2001 Park Nicollet Health*Source*®, Minneapolis, US.
Reprinted with permission.

Physical Activity and Your Child's Safety

Do you live in a neighborhood where you aren't comfortable having your child play outdoors unsupervised? These days, millions of parents feel this way. They're convinced that it simply isn't safe for their youngsters to be active outdoors, particularly on their own. And if parents are working during the day, it's not surprising that they don't want their youngsters spending time outside when they're not home.

One of the best options for you to explore is whether there's a formal after-school program in your neighborhood in which your child can participate that involves physical activity. For example, call the YMCA in your community, or the Boys & Girls Club. Enroll your child in a dance class to learn jazz or tap. Support your child in joining a youth bowling league. Be on the lookout for activities that are available in your community that include boys and girls. Remember that participation is the key. Your child will be supervised while staying active, and you can pick him up on the way home from work. Keeping him busy after school is the key to making sure he stays away from the television set.

If your youngster is old enough to stay home by himself in the afternoons until you return from work, help him plan that time in advance. He doesn't have to watch TV, play video games, or eat. In fact, there are many ways in which your child can stay active indoors. Sit down with him and let him choose some after-school activities such as

- Dancing to his favorite music on the CD player or tape deck
- Jumping rope

- Spending a few minutes with an exercise bike or treadmill (if you have either)
- Doing some chores that you assign him—from cleaning up his room to emptying the dishwasher
- Turning on a children's exercise video and working out for 30 minutes

Many children are more likely to put an exercise video into the VCR or DVD player if siblings or parents can work out with them. They may simply find it more fun to participate in physical activity with someone else. So if your child has brothers or sisters, get them involved as much as possible.

What Does Your Child's School Offer?

When you were in school, was physical education (PE)—or recess—your favorite "class"?

In many US schools, things have changed. Primarily because of budget cuts, PE programs have been sacrificed. Most states no longer mandate that their public schools offer PE. In some schools, PE classes are limited to once or twice a week, or they've been eliminated completely. Children are paying the price.

As we've emphasized in this chapter, physical activity is crucial to your child's health and the management of his weight. If your youngster's school district has reduced or eliminated PE programs, you need to let the district know that you want these classes back. Tell your child's school principal. Write a letter to the members of the local school board. If you and other parents raise your voices, it might make a difference.

Finding Time to Be Active

See if this scenario sounds familiar—your child has come home from school with 2 hours of homework, including studying for a math test the following day. He also needs to start working on a science fair project. And don't forget the clarinet lesson that's on his calendar as well. There seems to be barely enough time to fit in dinner and a bath.

No wonder some kids feel that they just don't have time for physical activity. Their schedules are filled to overflowing, and when they're overbooked, it's easy for physical activity to fall by the wayside.

As a parent, you need to intervene to make sure your child has time for all the things that are important. Whether he's overweight, physical activity needs to be a priority.

Sit down with your child and structure his time after school so he can fit in everything that's most essential. For example, in planning the following day, you might say something like, "You have a block of after-school time tomorrow. Maybe the time immediately after school isn't the best time for homework, because it will take up the daylight hours you could be outside playing. Why don't you think about choosing to play outdoors for 30 minutes or an hour after you get home? Then we'll go to your clarinet lesson, and once you've eaten dinner and it's dark outside, you can do your homework. The evening is the time when you used to watch TV anyway, so it's a good time to get your homework done. And let's think about rescheduling your clarinet lessons for the weekends."

As a parent, you can help your child find the opportunities to be active. If you're creative, the time will almost always be there.

Turning Family Time Into Active Time

For a lot of families, Sunday afternoons are a time to be together at the movies or the mall. As enjoyable as those outings may be, start thinking about spending some of that family time doing physical activities that all of you like.

Some overweight children are so averse to exercising that the first step in the right direction needs to be taken with their families. They may feel much more comfortable being active with their parents and siblings than with their peers, at least to start with. So why not play catch in the backyard, or dust off the tennis rackets in the closet and spend an hour hitting a tennis ball at the neighborhood courts? Rather than going to the movies, take a family hike in the hills near your home. When the whole family is involved, your overweight child is more likely to join in. Once he starts losing weight and gets more accustomed to moving his body, he may be more willing to step out and join a swimming program at the YMCA or take karate lessons at the local martial arts studio.

Spend a few moments thinking of other activities that your entire family can do together. Remember, the activity should be fun. If you need some suggestions, why not consider the following?

- Go to the park and throw the football back and forth.
- Play tag in the front yard.
- Go to the community pool for a family swim.
- Buy a kite, put it together as a family activity, and fly it in the park. While you hold onto the kite string, let your child run with the kite until the wind catches it and sends it aloft.

- Take a family bike ride.
- Go horseback riding.
- Wax the car as a family activity.
- Go to the mall—not only to shop, and certainly not to spend time at the food court, but to walk from one end of the mall to the other.
- During the holiday season, take a family walk in the evening and enjoy the holiday lights on the homes in the neighborhood.

When you join in, your child will see that you believe physical activity is important, and you'll become his most important role model.

Talking With Your Pediatrician

How much does your child weigh? The higher the number on the scale, the greater the chance that he is out of shape or deconditioned.

Before your youngster moves from a sedentary to a more active way of life, and particularly if he has any health problems, talk to your pediatrician. Your pediatrician will be able to tell you how to ensure that exercising is a safe and enjoyable experience for your child. Above all, ask the pediatrician whether your child has any physical limitations that you need to keep in mind. For example, many parents think that youngsters who have asthma can't play outdoors on a cold day, or they'll risk having asthmatic episodes. Your pediatrician can help you and your child plan for safe outdoor activity by including this option in your child's asthma plan.

Looking Forward

In the months and years ahead, don't back away from your commitment to promote physical activity in your child's life. Encourage any form of exercise or other activity that he enjoys and is willing to do regularly. Not only will he be better able to successfully manage his weight, but he has a much greater likelihood of enjoying a healthy life well into and throughout adulthood.

Let's complete this chapter with an assessment of your child's physical activity.

WORKSHEET TO TAKE TO YOUR PEDIATRICIAN

#10: WHERE DOES YOUR CHILD STAND?

What's Currently Happening With Physical Activity?
Let's take a few moments to determine how your child is currently faring in terms of physical activity. The answers to the following questions will help you identify how much time your child spends in structured and unstructured activities and areas in which your child may need to improve.

How many days a week does your child participate in physical education (PE) classes at school? _____

On those days, approximately how many minutes does your child spend moving or doing activity (as opposed to standing around) in those PE classes? _____

How many days a week does your child play outdoors? _____

About how many minutes (or hours) does your child spend playing outdoors on a typical weekday? _____ On a typical Saturday or Sunday? _____

What structured physical activities does your child participate in (for example, a youth sports team or organized activities at an after-school program)?

_____

_____

In a typical week, how many minutes (or hours) does your child spend in these structured activities? _____

On average, how many hours a day does your child watch TV or play video or computer games? _____

Does your child often snack while in front of the TV or computer screen? _____

What outdoor physical activities does your child enjoy doing?

_____

_____

What other outdoor physical activities would you like to introduce to your child?

_____

_____

_____

(Worksheet continued on page 66)

What is Going Well?

Use the answers to the previous questions to determine those areas in which your child is already doing well incorporating physical activity in his or her life. In the following space, write down the ways in which your child is active:

_____

_____

_____

What Changes Need to Be Made?

Next, take a few minutes to determine areas in which your child needs to improve. For example,

Does your child need to spend more time playing outdoors? _____

Would your child benefit from participating in youth sports or other organized activities? Would your child get more benefit and be more successful with activities in a small group or with his family?

_____

Does your child need to spend less time in front of the TV or computer or playing video games? _____

Choose a way in which your child can become more active, and write down a strategy for incorporating that activity into his or her life. For example, you may feel your child is watching too much TV after school and explore after-school activities at the local YMCA or Boys & Girls Club. Or you may find that your child is more comfortable increasing activity with a family member by taking a walk or shooting some hoops with a sibling.

_____

_____

What additional improvements would you like to help your child make in his or her efforts to become more active?

_____

_____

_____

_____

4

Your Role as a Parent: Developing a Consistent Approach

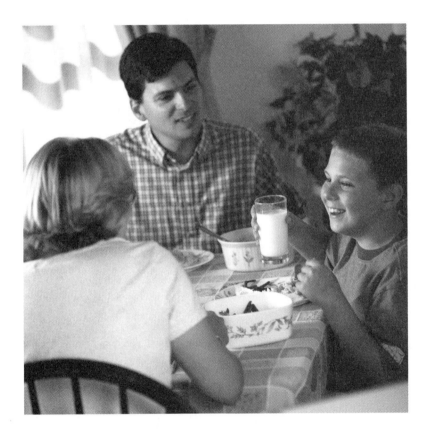

Parenting is filled with challenges. As your child grows from infancy through childhood, there is no one more important to her development than you. Not a day goes by when you're not called on to ensure her physical, emotional, social, and intellectual well-being.

If your child is overweight, however, you may feel that your parenting responsibilities have been turned up a notch. Almost by definition, weight management is a difficult challenge. As the primary person keeping your child consistently moving in the direction of steady weight loss—one meal or snack after another, one physical activity after the next—your challenges may seem daunting at times.

In this and the next 2 chapters, we'll equip you with information to help take much of the anxiety out of your parenting role. In the months and years ahead, the most important changes will start and continue at home with your family and child. We'll examine how your own parenting style may influence your child's success in her efforts at controlling her weight. You'll also find some concrete parenting guidance to help your child navigate the inevitable obstacles she'll encounter as she makes progress toward her goals.

Parents often say that they have difficulty keeping their children's eating and activity behaviors pointed in the right direction. Sometimes they may believe that they just don't have the skills to keep their families consistently on track. They simply might feel weary about making decisions, on almost an hour-by-hour basis, that can help their children lose weight. They might also find it difficult to deal with their children's complaints that they are no longer able to eat all the foods they want when they want, or that they are miserable because they can't watch TV all day on Saturday anymore. No wonder parents can feel exhausted.

Putting Health First

Do these scenarios sound familiar? Do you sometimes feel overwhelmed by the responsibilities of parenting an overweight youngster? Do you often feel that you're not up to the task, or does your child somehow make you feel heartless and mean-spirited when you insist on refocusing the family in a way that supports the loss of her excess weight?

Keep in mind that nearly every parent of an obese child feels exactly the same way from time to time. But don't lose your direction. You need to consistently think of your decisions in this area as more than weight-related decisions. You should start reframing them as *health-oriented,* not *weight-oriented* ones, and remember that improving your child's health is the ultimate goal. After all, as a parent, you're used to making health decisions for your family. You do it every day, and it's probably something that you've become very good at. For example, you don't have a problem making sure that your child gets all the vaccinations she needs, even when she complains that she doesn't want a shot today. If your 12-year-old were to tell you that one of the kids in the neighborhood is smoking cigarettes and she wants to try it, too, you wouldn't hesitate to say "no" in the most forceful way possible. Your child's health is a priority, and it's an area in which you've been making decisions without hesitation.

That's exactly the same approach you should use for your child's overweight problem. Remember, obesity is a threat to her health, increasing her risk of developing a long list of serious illnesses. She is more likely to have high blood pressure. She may become vulnerable to type 2 diabetes. Blood tests might show that she has elevated triglyceride levels or a problem with her liver. She could develop asthma or gallstones.

For these reasons, you shouldn't think twice about doing what it takes to get your child's overweight problem under control. As her parent, you're the protector of her well-being. It's one of your most important responsibilities. Each time you make a weight-related decision, it's as important as any other judgment about your family's health. You can't be passive when your child's health is at stake. By making the right decisions now, you'll be affecting her well-being far into the future.

You Are the Agent for Change

Earlier in the book, we described your child's efforts to lose weight as a journey. At times, it might seem like the journey is taking you and your youngster down a long and winding road where the results you're seeking are far off in the distance. As an adult and a parent, you are the person who needs to make sure that your overweight child and entire family stay the course. You are the captain of the ship that is helping your child navigate and surmount all the challenges that are ahead. *You are the agent for change.*

As you guide your child along the path toward a healthier weight, you need to stay a step ahead of her to keep her moving toward the destination. That means focusing some of your energy on establishing boundaries that set the stage for her success. Actually, this should be a familiar parental task because in one form or another, you've been doing it since your child was an infant. In the preschool years, for example, you taught her rules for negotiating her way successfully through the world she lives in—the importance of crossing streets only when the traffic signal is green, sharing toys with friends, and brushing her teeth before she goes to sleep. In the same way, you need to create boundaries and guidelines that will help her make healthy choices today.

Where should you begin? A good starting point is right at home. That means taking charge of the family's day-to-day environment. It means creating the conditions for change to take place, with minimal conflict or confrontation. It means eliminating as many temptations as possible.

In the previous chapters, we've already given you some ideas for seizing control of what goes on at home, from keeping unhealthy snacks out of the cupboard to taking the entire family on a walk after dinner rather than turning on the TV. It also means giving your child choices, but only within the limits of safe, healthy boundaries. For instance,

- You can provide the play equipment, and she can decide whether to jump rope or throw a ball against the garage door.
- You can invite her to help prepare her lunch, and let her choose from among several healthy entrees that you can make together.
- You can keep tempting high-calorie snack foods (cookies, candy bars) out of your grocery basket, and instead let her choose from among healthier alternatives that stock your kitchen cupboard.

Remember, your home environment is something that you can control almost completely. It gives you enormous power in becoming an agent for change and helping her successfully manage her obesity.

Customizing Approaches for Your Family

No two families are alike. What works for yours may send another family spinning out of the control, even when they're dealing with exactly the same issues. There is no single best way of managing a particular situation, so be willing to fine-tune the strategies you adopt until you're getting the job done.

Of course, you need to identify the changes you want and what may be getting in the way of those changes being made, particularly over the long term (self-assessment should help you do that). If your child overdoes the afternoon snacking when she gets home from school, maybe you need to limit the time she has available for indulging in these munchies. Keep her attention directed elsewhere, perhaps having her play outside with friends immediately after school or getting her involved in an after-school activity.

Not surprisingly, your parental interventions may evolve as your child gets older. You can't expect the same approaches that worked when she was 8 years old to still work at 14 years. As a teenager, if she'd prefer to sit at the computer for hours after school, exchanging instant messages with her friends and eating all the while, you're not going to necessarily be able to send her outside to the neighborhood playground with swings and monkey bars. But you can explore other activities that will keep her busy. How about encouraging your adolescent to volunteer at the public library, helping out at the pre-schoolers' story hour? Or why not sign her up for an ice skating class or tennis lessons? Or maybe she can try out for the school softball team. In virtually every community, there are plenty of healthy after-school options.

Whatever your child decides to do, you need to monitor her consistently. Many parents assume that once their youngsters reach a certain age, they'll know what to do to stay active, or they'll instinctively choose a healthier snack over a less healthy one. Not true. Every child can use some help and support. For that reason, don't

Setting Shorter Term, Achievable Goals

If your child is determined to lose weight, have the two of you (along with your pediatrician) discussed a weight-loss strategy? No matter how ambitious the goal, it's important that you encourage her to set some shorter term goals that she can reach along the way that will keep her motivated to stay the course.

Use this same approach in every aspect of this program. Guide your child toward deciding what she wants to achieve, and then help her get there in small steps. If she needs to spend more time being physically active, perhaps start with just a few minutes of outdoor play after school and build on that.

See yourself as a parental support system. Help your youngster set short-term goals and make small changes that can add up to big improvements. If those goals involve reducing her time in front of the TV and becoming more physically active, they'll become an important way for the entire family to move a step closer to a healthier lifestyle.

leave these decisions solely in your child's hands. You're still the parent, and you're a full partner in this change that your child is making. It's your parental responsibility to make sure she keeps moving in the direction of better health.

The Power of Family

Imagine your overweight child sitting on the couch along with the entire family, watching a rented movie. But while everyone else is munching on cookies in front of the TV, she's trying to restrain herself from reaching for a handful of her own. It's a bit of torture that is setting her up for failure.

Without a doubt, it is much easier to make changes when those around you are adopting the same new behaviors as you. As we'll emphasize throughout this book, your child's success in losing weight is dependent on the support of the entire family—parents, partners, siblings, grandparents, uncles, aunts, cousins, and anyone else who spends time with her. Part of your parenting responsibility is to let the other adults in your child's life (schoolteachers, church leaders, scoutmasters, relatives) know about your child's efforts so they won't undermine them. All it takes are a few acts of sabotage, however innocent or unintentional, to tip your youngster in the wrong direction and derail weeks of her best efforts.

At every opportunity, your family needs to demonstrate support for your overweight youngster. You need to be consistent in approaching your child's weight problem because you have the primary responsibility for managing her nutrition and physical activity. If you're divorced from your child's other parent, you need to share information with your former spouse on an ongoing basis. You need to mutually decide on any changes in the environment that need to be made at each of your respective homes. Even when you're divorced, you need to close ranks and stand together in every aspect of parenting.

Structured Eating

As you might guess, when you have a child trying to lose weight, you need to pay particular attention to mealtimes. They should be firmly structured, not only for your obese youngster, but for the entire family. In general, 3 meals and 1 to 2 snacks per day, without any meal skipping, are optimal (if your child skips a meal, she'll become over-hungry and set herself up for overeating). Also, if she knows that dinner is going to be served at 6:00 pm, she'll be less likely to start searching for a snack at 5:30 pm, whereas if dinner is served at a different time every night (for example, sometimes at 6:00 pm, but other times at 8:00 pm), she might grab a snack at 5:30 pm rather than risk having to wait 2 or 3 hours for her hunger pangs to be satisfied.

There's another very important element to structured eating, and that's ensuring that the family eats together as often as possible with no distractions. In too many homes, families rarely sit down for a meal together, and when they do, the TV is on and no one (except maybe for a sitcom star or the local newscaster) says a word throughout the dinner hour. The TV is a disruption that you should avoid while you're eating.

Just how important are family meals? In many households, they're the only period of the day when the family is together, giving every adult and child an opportunity to talk about what happened at school or work. It's a time when the family can grow closer to one another. It's also a time to teach your child about healthy, balanced meals and optimal portion sizes and when you can serve as a role model for healthy eating. You can also offer encouragement to your

Weekend Perils

Some parents feel they've got good control over how their children's lives unfold during the week. There's a structure to the day, Monday through Friday, incorporating school and extracurricular activities, that helps them effectively manage their children's nutrition and activity levels.

Then the weekend arrives. The routine that they relied on during the previous 5 days simply isn't there, and that's when trouble often rises to the surface. On Saturdays, the kids might end up watching TV from sunup to exhaustion (if you let them). In the process, they're not getting any exercise, and they're probably overindulging on snacks when they're not playing with the remote control. Then there are the weekend dinners at the family's favorite all-you-can-eat restaurant, or the afternoon at the baseball stadium where everyone has one hot dog too many.

What's the solution? Saturdays and Sundays need to be planned as carefully as the rest of your child's week. Help schedule her time so that at least part of every Saturday and Sunday is devoted to physical activity. Sign her up for a Saturday afternoon sports program at the community center. At home, make sure that only healthy snacks are available for her to grab. There's no need for your child to backslide on the weekends, but it will take some consistent parental planning to ensure that it doesn't happen.

youngster, celebrate her successes, and reassure her if she's having difficulties. As an added benefit, you'll be able to keep an eye on what and how much she is eating.

One other note—these family meals will probably become less common as your child enters adolescence. Once she's involved in rehearsals for the high school play or is gone because of a part-time job at the local pharmacy, you'll covet those days when the family could be together at the dinner table. Treat these opportunities as precious moments that will become some of your sweetest family memories many years down the road.

Partnering With Your Pediatrician

Since the time your child was born, you have relied on your pediatrician to play multiple roles in your youngster's life, from providing physical examinations to treating her illnesses to administering her immunizations on schedule. Don't overlook the important supportive role your pediatrician can play by partnering with your family in your child's weight-loss efforts.

Each time you visit the pediatrician's office, particularly for scheduled checkups, your doctor or a nurse will weigh and measure your youngster and calculate her body mass index. He or she will check her overall health status and monitor any obesity-related health conditions she may have, such as high blood pressure or high cholesterol levels.

Your pediatrician can also talk to your child about her weight problem at a level appropriate for her age. The doctor can help you and your youngster prioritize the changes that need to be made first

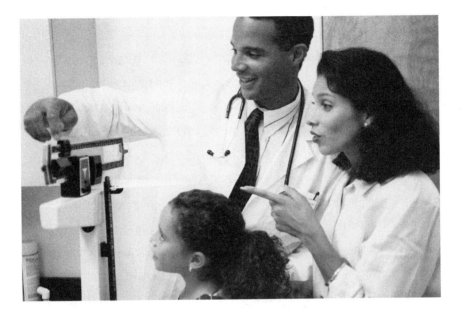

to get her weight problem under control and help you set some health goals, including lifestyle changes such as eating more healthfully, becoming more physically active, and watching less TV.

Also, turn to your child's pediatrician for guidance on child development issues. The doctor can answer questions like, "At my child's age, what is she capable of doing on her own as we're adopting a more healthful lifestyle?" As you might guess, and your pediatrician can help explain, a 14-year-old is able to do much more than a 4-year-old. It isn't developmentally appropriate, for example, to put your 4-year-old in charge of getting her own snacks from the refrigerator and expect her to make appropriate choices, but a 14-year-old who you've educated about healthy snacking might be trusted to do so.

The Community and Schools

Your parenting responsibilities extend far beyond what's happening in your home. Your child spends plenty of time at school and perhaps a child care center, and as we've emphasized elsewhere in this book, you need to make sure that the foods she eats are healthy and compatible with the nutritional plan that she's following at home. In chapters 2 and 3, we emphasized the importance of gathering information about school menus, learning what your child is being fed at child care, and asking how much physical activity she's getting. If you're not pleased with the answers you're getting—perhaps your child's school has phased out recess or serves too many high-fat, high-calorie foods and snacks without much nutritional value in the cafeteria or student store—you need to raise your voice and request changes. If your child is in preschool, talk to the teachers and ask for healthier snacks. You might find that your child's teacher will actively become an ally in supporting your child's weight-loss efforts.

Recruit other parents to join you and raise your voices in unison. In the best-case scenario, your school administrators will reassess what they're doing and make changes toward better nutrition for the entire school. If change isn't forthcoming, start packing a sack lunch for your child as a way to ensure that she'll get the kind of healthy nourishment she needs.

Keeping Focused on the Goal

Particularly in a book about overweight children, it might be easy to become preoccupied with the kinds and amounts of food that your youngster eats. Of course, we're not saying that your child's nutrition isn't important—in fact, we devoted Chapter 2 to it. Even so, there are other significant topics that deserve your attention as well.

Much of your focus as a parent should be on changing your child's behavior and lifestyle. It should be on consistently living a *healthier* life. As we'll emphasize throughout this book, the weight will come off if you and your child are making healthy choices. In essence, her weight will take care of itself. Once you let go of your preoccupation with your child's weight, it will free you to handle

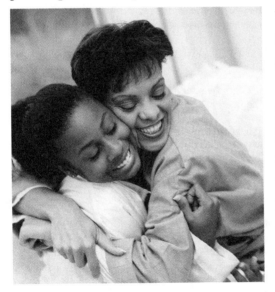

what needs to be done to ensure her overall good health.

Remember, you and your youngster are on a journey that, like any trip, requires a plan and clear vision of your destination. Remind her that you're on this journey toward better health together, every step of the way.

WORKSHEET TO TAKE TO YOUR PEDIATRICIAN

#11: ASSESSING YOUR HOME ENVIRONMENT

Let's continue the journey toward helping your child manage his or her weight by pausing at this checkpoint to make another assessment. This time, you'll evaluate the following components of this part of the road trip toward controlling his obesity:

- Your home environment
- Your parenting role within this environment
- Areas in which improvements may be needed

What Is Currently Happening at Home?
In answering the following questions, you'll get a clearer sense of what is taking place in your home environment that may play a role in your youngster's health.

Does your family mostly eat well-balanced meals? During a typical week, how many well-balanced meals are prepared in the home?

Breakfast _____   Lunch _____   Dinner _____

On average, how many times a week does the family eat fast-food meals that are brought into the home or eaten at restaurants? _____

Who does the grocery shopping in your family? _____

Do other family members (for example, parents, children) contribute to the decisions on what will be purchased in the supermarket? If so, who? Is most of the food brought into the home healthy? _____

Who is giving your child snacks at home (or elsewhere)?
- ☐ Parent(s)
- ☐ Other family members
- ☐ Other children
- ☐ Child care staff

Does your overweight child and/or family use food
- ☐ As a reward?
- ☐ For comfort?
- ☐ To relieve boredom?

Is your child physically active every day? _____

How much time does your child spend in physical activities each day? _____

How many hours do family members spend watching TV or on the computer every day? _____

How many TVs/computers do you have in the house? _____

Do family members have TVs/computers in their bedrooms? _____

Does your child have a TV/computer in his or her bedroom? _____

Who sets limits on your child's TV/computer use? _____

How many hours does your child watch TV or play computer or video games during a typical day? _____

What Is Going Well in Your Household?
Based on your previous answers, what areas are you pleased with in your home life that contribute to your child's health? Specifically, check off what is going well in your household.

- ☐ Well-balanced meals
- ☐ Healthy snacking
- ☐ Limiting fast-food meals
- ☐ Regularly participating in physical activity
- ☐ Limiting TV watching and video or computer games

Use this space to elaborate on any of the above:

_____

_____

What Problems Exist in Your Household?
What problem areas are present in your home environment that may need changing or improving (place a check mark by those that apply)?

- ☐ Poor food/meal selection
- ☐ Poor snack food choices
- ☐ Too many fast-food meals
- ☐ Not enough physical activity or time outdoors
- ☐ Too much computer, TV, or video game time

Others: _____

_____

What Change(s) Do You Need to Make and How Will You Make Them?
As the next step in your journey toward better health, identify the specific obstacles that are contributing to your household problems. Which of the following apply to you and your family?

- ☐ Family preferences (for example, unhealthy favorite foods)
- ☐ Not enough available time (to prepare meals, for physical activity)
- ☐ Not enough money
- ☐ Not enough time spent outdoors
- ☐ No safe places to play
- ☐ Your child won't go to activities or play outside
- ☐ Other

(Worksheet continued on page 84)

Next, select a single, specific change that you'd like to work on with your child and the rest of the family (for example, improving the snacks available in your house and chosen by your family).

_____

_____

To make this change possible, identify who can support you in this process. In addition to your and your child, who else can go on this journey with you, and can help your child reach this goal?

- ☐ Your spouse
- ☐ Your other children
- ☐ Grandparents
- ☐ Others

Now, use the following space to create a plan to make possible the change you've chosen.

_____

_____

In the past, how has your child reacted and how did you respond to your child when you tried to make changes (for example, did you give in to your child's complaints or demands)?

_____

_____

What could you do differently this time? How can you change your own actions to produce more positive results?

_____

_____

From a parenting point of view, is there anything else standing in the way of making healthier changes in your home environment?

_____

_____

_____

_____

5

What's Your Parenting Style? Assessing Your Strengths and Challenges

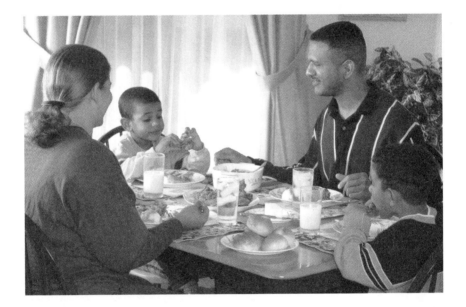

If your child is going to succeed at losing weight, that effort needs to begin at home. The way your youngster eats starts right in your own kitchen. The choices he makes to become active may begin with a conversation over the dinner table and lead to the parks and playgrounds in your own neighborhood.

In these parenting chapters, you'll learn that your skills, style, and decisions as a parent clearly matter where your child's weight is concerned. At the same time, for most parents, even those who are (or once had been) overweight themselves, this may still seem like largely uncharted territory. After all, helping a child reach his weight-loss goals and fully understanding the parent-child dynamics that can contribute to his success or setbacks aren't taught in most parenting books and classes. In this chapter and the one that follows, we'll help you examine and more fully appreciate how you and the entire family contribute to your child's ability to lose weight. As you'll read, you can help him see the importance of adopting healthy habits that can last a lifetime. On the other hand, you might use food in a negative way (as a reward, for example) that could undermine your child's hope of successful weight loss. We'll even explore how your own childhood experiences, including the messages you got from your own parents about food and weight, may be a factor in how you and your child relate to each other about this issue.

As we'll emphasize throughout this book, a balanced diet and regular physical activity can promote good health in your child. But meaningful change will happen only if you're willing to work with him in taking small steps forward that can make a big difference in his well-being and weight.

Your Own Family Background

Understanding yourself as a parent starts with looking at your own family when you were growing up. Parents often react to their own childhood experiences by either trying to reproduce them or trying not to make the same mistakes. Either way, it is important to know where you came from to plan where you are going.

Let's begin by examining your own childhood and the relationship that you've had to food and body weight. By answering these questions thoughtfully, you may gain some insights into your current thinking about your child's food intake and his obesity.

You (and your spouse or your child's other parent) should consider these questions and review your answers together. You might find some similarities in your backgrounds—or some marked differences that could contribute to conflicts or problems in the way each of you approaches your child's excess weight.

- When you were growing up, did your family life tend to revolve around food and meals? _____
  - What about at family gatherings and holidays? _____
- At mealtimes, was there always plenty of food on the dining room table? _____
- Did your parent(s) place serving dishes on the dinner table so you could easily help yourself to seconds and choose your own portion sizes? _____
  - Did you often take seconds? _____

- Did your parent(s) usually insist that you eat everything on your plate, even when you were no longer hungry? _____
- Were you overweight as a child?
  - If "yes," do you think your excess weight changed your life in any major way? _____ If so, how? _____
- Did you often try to lose weight as a child? _____
  - Were those efforts successful? _____
  - Were they ever a source of conflict between you and your parents? _____
- Were your mother and/or father overweight? _____
- Were your grandparents overweight? _____
- As a child, were you often preoccupied with thoughts of food during the day? _____
- Did you eat secretly so your parent(s) and other family members wouldn't know how much you ate? _____
  - If "yes," how often did you eat this way (for example, daily, weekly)? _____
- During your childhood, did your parent(s) sometimes use food as
  - A reward? _____
  - A bribe? _____
  - A source of comfort? _____
- Were you physically active with regularity as a child? _____
  - In school? _____
  - Outside of school? _____
  - In youth sports (for example, soccer, Little League)? _____

■ What types of activities did you participate in?

_____

_____

_____

■ Did your family participate in physical activities together? _____
■ What types of physical activities did you do as a family? _____
■ If you could change anything about your childhood (as it relates to the issues mentioned herein), what would you change? _____

_____

_____

■ How do you think your own childhood experiences with food and physical activity influence the way you're raising your own child today?

_____

_____

_____

Did some of these questions strike a chord with you? In many cultures, for example, food is a very important part of family life. When extended families get together, much of the attention seems to focus on large, high-calorie meals, and as a result, the waistlines of everyone at the dinner table often pay the price.

On the other hand, perhaps you grew up in a family for which money was scarce and there wasn't a lot of extra food for second helpings—or sometimes even first helpings! These are experiences that will linger with you for a lifetime, and when you have children of your own, you might think, "It's important for me to make sure my children will always have *all* the food they want."

As you contemplate the answers to these questions, think back to the worksheet you filled out in Chapter 1 that evaluated your family's health history, including whether you, your spouse or your child's other parent, and other family members have had obesity-related chronic health problems over the years, including heart disease, high cholesterol levels, diabetes, and asthma. These medical histories can provide clues to your own child's risks and should motivate you to work hard to help your youngster manage his own weight, thus reducing his likelihood of developing chronic illnesses now and in the future.

Use the answers in worksheet #1 as a springboard for family discussion, and help everyone understand what may be driving some of your own concerns about your child's weight and how you're trying to deal with them. Maybe you grew up with parents who told you to eat everything on your plate, perhaps using the logic that there were "children starving in China." As an adult, you know the perils of prompting your youngster to continue eating even after he's full; if you do it routinely, it can deliver a knockout blow to all of your positive efforts at encouraging weight loss. By sharing the experiences of your own childhood, you may better understand some of the issues that have arisen in your family life today.

Putting Food in Perspective

As important as it is to pay attention to the dietary and lifestyle changes that can help your child successfully manage his weight, don't become overfocused on them, particularly your child's food choices.

If you were overweight yourself when you were his age, you might feel that you'll do whatever it takes to help him avoid the same emotional pain that you went through. But some parents become obsessed with the food their children are consuming. They spend most of their mealtimes together—and just about every other available moment—talking with their children about what they're eating or shouldn't be eating. They discuss calories, portion sizes, and fat content. They feed on the latest news about fad diets. You'd think there was nothing else going on in their children's worlds.

There is such an overemphasis on food in some families that it gets in the way of having a balanced relationship between parents and children. Remember, there's more to your youngster's life than what he's eating and how much he weighs. (How about asking, "What did you do at school today?" or "How much homework do you have tonight?") By keeping food in perspective and focusing on the rest of your child's interests and activities, you can make mealtime a positive time for both of you.

Family Interactions

The support your child needs to steadily and successfully lose weight should be a family affair. As you've read in earlier chapters, your obese youngster needs the entire family to get onboard—parents, grandparents, brothers, and sisters—and unanimously agree to keep foods like potato chips and chocolate chip cookies out of the house and get more physical activity, even among those who have no excess weight to lose.

Keep in mind that as a parent, you want *all* of your children to live a life of optimal health, no matter what their weights. You want their hearts to stay healthy. You want their blood pressure to stay normal. You want them to avoid diabetes. For that reason, this is an important and even exciting journey for the family to embark on, and although you're the tour guide on this trip, it's one that the whole family needs to take together. Everyone should sign on as a demonstration of support for your obese child—and in the process, they'll improve their own well-being, as well.

Over the ensuing weeks and months, you should have regular family meetings. Discuss how everyone is doing on this mission to better health. What has been the hardest part for everyone? What was the most difficult change to make, and what was easier than anyone had imagined? Are all family members on board with these changes? What still needs to be done? Also make sure that the family understands that almost inevitably, there will be ups and downs in this journey.

At times, an older overweight child may feel guilty if he plateaus and seems to be getting nowhere in his weight-loss efforts, or perhaps he'll regain some of the weight he had lost. He might even become the target of blame or anger from siblings who feel he hasn't been trying hard enough. Explain that pointing fingers only gets in the way of progress. As long as there's internal bickering and family members who are playing the blame game, it's virtually impossible for your obese youngster to move forward again.

Is Divorce Part of Your Family's Reality?

If you and your spouse are divorced, both of you should work extra hard to make sure you remain active players in your overweight child's support team. Take responsibility for maintaining the healthiest possible home environment. Make sure it's as conducive as possible to helping your child reach his weight-loss goals.

Even if you and your child's other parent don't see eye to eye on everything, your youngster's well-being should be an area where you can come together. Nevertheless, getting both parents and other family members to participate actively in the child's weight-loss program doesn't always happen. In some families, only one parent recognizes that the youngster's weight is a problem; the other parent, particularly if this parent never had a weight problem of his or her own, might have a "What's the big deal?" attitude and may not understand how hard it can be to lose weight.

If you're frustrated because your former spouse isn't as interested in this family journey as you are, do the best you can. Take charge of what takes place in your own home when your child is there. That's what you should focus on. Continue to encourage your ex-spouse to make changes for the sake of your youngster, without assigning blame or perhaps making matters worse. Eventually, your spouse may decide to change course for the good of the family.

Emotions and Food

Children (as well as adults) use food for reasons other than to satisfy their hunger and nutritional needs. In fact, obese youngsters often eat in response to their emotions and feelings. For example, at the beginning of this chapter, we raised the issue of whether your own parents used food for comfort in your household. This is a common phenomenon, beginning at birth. A baby's crying or irritability is typically met with breast milk or infant formula, and feeding becomes a way of calming and quieting him. At birthdays and holidays, when children are surrounded by family and are feeling loved, they're often given cookies or other desserts that become a symbol of this love and caring.

These days, whenever your own child is feeling anxious, perhaps related to an upcoming math test or because he's being teased at school, he may turn back to food as one way of making him feel better. At the same time, however, there are many other reasons beyond comfort that may prompt children to eat. For example, does your youngster sometimes reach for food when he's experiencing any of the following?

- Boredom
- Insecurity
- Anger
- Depression
- Loneliness
- Happiness
- Stress
- Fatigue
- Frustration
- Resentment

Even though food can become a welcome companion for your child, the outcome may not be quite what he expected. Ironically, if he overeats as a way to soften feelings of insecurity or depression, for instance, or perhaps because of stress over an oral report he needs to give at school, he may feel even worse after a food binge, knowing that it can aggravate his weight problem. Before the food is even digested, he might be feeling guilt or shame.

In fact, one of your biggest parenting challenges is for you and your child to determine whether he's eating for the right reasons. Ask yourself questions like, does he eat at times other than regular mealtimes and snacks? Is he munching at every opportunity? What factors might be contributing to his overeating that call for you to intervene?

Some parents inadvertently contribute to their children's obesity by rewarding their youngsters with food (does an A on a test sometimes lead to a trip to the ice cream shop?). There are other, healthier ways to offer praise and rewards. For a young child, how about giving him a few stickers as a reward, or perhaps schedule a shopping trip to buy a toy or new pair of shoes?

Don't overlook the importance of verbal praise. When your child is doing things right, tell him. Notice how words of approval can boost his self-esteem and help keep him motivated to continue making the right decisions for his health and weight. Even when he's having difficulties staying on course with his diet, look for other ways to offer praise ("You walked more than half a mile today, that's so great!"). When he backslides, don't nag him or make him feel like he has failed. Encourage him to keep moving forward, and even if he complains from time to time ("I want a soft drink, not ice water"), encourage him to stay the course. Offer him all the support he needs and deserves.

It's important for parents to listen to how they're speaking to their children. Is it mostly negative? Is it often critical? It's hard for anyone, including children, to make changes in that kind of environment. Some parents actually try to embarrass their overweight children into making changes ("Billy, you're getting fatter again!"), figuring that if he sees himself as unsightly, he'll be motivated to lose weight. Don't count on that strategy working. Even if your child is able to make changes under these circumstances, those improvements are not likely to last without some parental praise and positive reinforcement along the way.

Equal Versus Equality

The goals for diet and physical activity should be different for a 10-year-old than a 5-year-old, taking into account their different developmental stages. Your children, however, may not see it that way. At the dinner table, your 5-year-old daughter might say that she wants to eat the same amounts of food as her older sister. You need to explain that their ages and stages are different. Yes, you will treat them with equality, but that doesn't mean that they'll receive equal portion sizes or that you'll challenge them to exercise in exactly the same way. Paying attention to each individual child's needs for rightsized nutrition and activity is more easily done at home than when you eat out.

Of course, if you frequently eat out at restaurants, you've certainly noticed that portions these days are likely to be enormous in size. Restaurant chefs seem to think that the more calories they provide, the happier their customers will be. Maybe so, but that approach can rapidly undermine your child's efforts to eat less than he used to. While overeating isn't inevitable at a restaurant, it's much more likely when plates are filled to overflowing. Those kinds of temptations can be hard to resist.

That's why when weight loss is a goal for one or more family members, consider eating most of your meals at home, where you'll have better control of the amounts of food that end up on the dining room table. When the family

(continued on page 98)

eats dinner together, you can prepare the same foods for everyone, perhaps giving all the children servings of chicken, vegetables, and potatoes, along with a glass of milk. You shouldn't be serving your 8-year-old and 4-year-old the identical portion sizes, though. The portions on their plates should be age appropriate.

As we pointed out in Chapter 4, you'll also probably find that when the family sits down for a meal together, good things happen. According to the American Academy of Pediatrics, children who eat meals with their families are likely to consume more vegetables and fruits and less fried foods and soft drinks than children who eat less frequently with their families. It's another good reason to turn mealtime into family time.

Important Points to Remember

- Your own relationship with food and weight, dating back to your childhood, can influence the way you parent your own overweight youngster.
- Your obese child needs the support of your entire family. All family members should participate in the journey to better health.
- Provide your overweight child with plenty of parental praise and positive reinforcement, but don't reward your youngster with food.
- Finger-pointing gets in the way of progress toward weight loss and better health.
- Divorced parents should both take responsibility for maintaining the healthiest possible environment in their own homes.
- Keep your child's weight problem in perspective. There's more to your relationship with him than the number on the bathroom scale.

Time for Reevaluation

Next, let's pose some of the same questions we asked at the beginning of this chapter, and some additional ones, too—but this time, we'll highlight those that apply to your role as a parent or are relevant to your family life today. Even though you've already thought about some of these topics in earlier chapters of this book (like questions about your child's eating habits and activity level), reemphasizing them here can help you more fully understand the family dynamics that contribute to your child's obesity and help you in the journey toward better health on which your family is embarking. You'll see what you're doing right, as well as where you might need to improve.

No matter how you answer these questions, one thing is certain— you're reading this book because you care deeply about the well-being of your overweight child. You want the best for him, including as healthy a life as possible. If there are moments when you or your youngster feel discouraged, don't give up. Move past those negative thoughts. Be patient. This is a long-term adventure; it was never designed as a quick fix or a rapid over-and-done process.

Continue to teach your family a healthier way of life. Keep making small changes and over time, they'll make a big difference in your youngster's health. Remember, making reasonable changes is a reasonable thing to do where your child's health is concerned.

In the next chapter, we'll describe in detail some common trouble areas that you could encounter on this journey, from children who sneak food to cultural issues that can influence what your youngster eats. Chapter 6 will equip you with some tools and suggestions for continuing to move forward toward your child's weight-loss goals.

WORKSHEET TO TAKE TO YOUR PEDIATRICIAN
#12: TIME FOR REEVALUATION

What's Currently Happening?
Do your family life and schedule tend to revolve around food and meals?

Explain:

Is there always plenty of food on the dining room table?

Do you place serving dishes on the table so everyone can help themselves to seconds and choose their own portion sizes?

How often do family members reach for seconds?

Do you usually insist that your child eat everything on his plate, even when he or she is no longer hungry?

Is food an important part of large family gatherings and holidays?

What Is Going Well?
Have your child's eating habits changed in a positive way in recent days and weeks, based in part on the information you learned in Chapter 2 and elsewhere in this book?

What major changes have you already made?

Have you followed your pediatrician's advice on what your child should be eating?

What changes have you made in response to your pediatrician's guidance?

_____

Does your family do physical activities together?

_____

What activities does your family enjoy doing together?

_____

What Problems Still Exist?
Does your child sometimes seem to become preoccupied with thoughts of food during the day?

_____

Are you aware of whether your child eats secretly so you and other family members won't know how much he or she eats?

_____

Do you sometimes give your child mixed messages about the right foods to eat (for example, do you serve a salad for lunch, but then bake 2 dozen cookies and leave them on the kitchen counter where your child can get to them without you knowing)?

_____

Do you hide food for yourself so your child won't eat it (perhaps concealing it in your bedroom or on a high cupboard shelf in the kitchen)?

_____

In relating to your overweight child, do you sometimes use food as a

- ☐ Reward?
- ☐ Bribe?
- ☐ Source of comfort?

Has your child's level of physical activity changed, based in part on the information you read in Chapter 3 and guidance from your pediatrician?

_____

In what types of physical activity does your child now participate?

_____

_____

_____

(Worksheet continued on page 102)

What Changes Need to Be Made and How Will You Make Them?

Based on your answers to these questions, what areas related to your child's health still need improvement?

- ☐ Nutrition
- ☐ Physical activity
- ☐ TV/video game/computer time

What obstacles still exist that interfere with dealing effectively with these problems?

_____

_____

Do you use the TV as a babysitter, keeping your child occupied while you're busy doing something else?

_____

Choose one of the lifestyle changes listed previously that you haven't worked on yet. In the space below, describe in detail how you and the family plan to approach this problem in the days ahead.

_____

_____

_____

_____

Who can support you along the path toward change?

_____

_____

_____

_____

6

Parenting Challenges:
Working With Your Child to Get
Back to Good Health

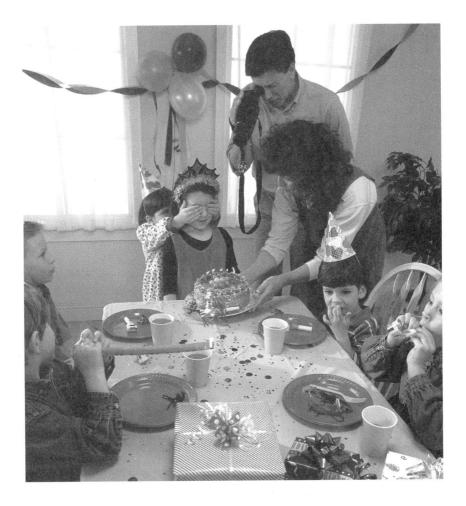

*E*ven though you and your family may be fully committed to helping your child try new foods, eat more fruits and vegetables, try healthier snacks, and exercise more, many challenges can still arise on this journey. If you are still thinking about helping your child with her weight, but are not sure if you are ready to start, don't stop reading. Spending time to get prepared to make change is important. Continue reading, jot down thoughts and questions, and talk with other family members and your child's pediatrician to get support. In fact, it's unrealistic to think that problems won't develop that require your attention and action. There may be plenty of obstacles along the way that could temporarily derail your youngster from the path toward better health.

In this chapter, we'll describe some of the most common challenges that you're likely to encounter. We'll discuss setbacks and backsliding, which are almost inevitable as you travel this road. You'll also read about other relevant issues that may apply to your child, from sneaking food to being teased and bullied. We'll also examine ways you can intervene to keep your child moving forward. Sometimes when setbacks happen, parents feel frustrated and may begin to bargain, cajole, and just plain focus on what's not happening with food and activity. This is tempting, but remember that your job is to provide good nutrition in proper portions to your child and family and then let them decide how much of that portion to eat and to encourage activity in a positive way. Staying positive and focusing on what's going right and all the other aspects of your child's life can help keep nutrition and activity change moving along.

Managing Setbacks and Detours

No matter how strong your child's determination is to gain better control over her food and activity choices, she'll probably experience some backsliding from time to time. Maybe she'll overeat for several days in a row. She might grab some unhealthy foods in the school cafeteria when she's feeling stressed about upcoming final examinations. Perhaps she'll attend a birthday party and help herself to more than one very large slice of cake—with extra ice cream on top.

As discouraged as you and your child might feel at those moments, you need to keep these lapses in perspective. You don't have to view them as the start down a slippery slope from which there's no turning back. Instead, think of them as just minor stumbling blocks, which is exactly what they are. Even if they add a pound or two to your child's weight, they're certainly not a reason for her to give up and abandon all the successes she's had so far. Remember that you are helping your child develop lifelong habits for healthy eating and activity. Learning how to make wise health decisions about nutrition and activity is what's important. Help your child learn that all-or-nothing thinking gets in the way of making changes and can lead to a pattern of restriction and overindulgence that not only doesn't feel good, but reinforces negative eating and activity patterns. Remember too, that when you let your child in on meal planning, food shopping and preparation, and planning family activities, she will learn to make good decisions from your example.

In fact, backsliding is a normal part of making any type of change. The key is not to get dejected. Instead, you and your child need to rethink what may have gone wrong and how you can minimize the risk of it happening again.

The first step in this process is to acknowledge that a setback has actually occurred or is still underway. Has your child stopped playing outdoors? Is she spending more time in front of the TV? Has the entire family started eating at fast-food restaurants more often than usual?

Once you give some thought to what might be going awry, the best corrections for your course may become rather obvious. Even so, you'd be surprised at how often parents and children know that something isn't going right, but never take the time to evaluate what's really happening. That's why it might be helpful to write down what your child is eating and what her activity level is. The mere act of putting this information down on paper can help you identify specific problem areas and when and why they might be taking place.

Are the setbacks occurring when grandma comes for a visit, for example? Does she bring some sweets with her that aren't ordinarily available in your home? Did your youngster go out for pizza or fast food 3 times last week, even though the family has been trying to stick to a once-a-week limit? Did you stop at the supermarket on the way home from work twice in recent days and buy some soda for the entire family to grab? Does it follow periods of abstinence or withholding foods?

No matter what the problems are, they're now in the past. Rather than becoming frustrated or perhaps even scolding your child or other family members for these inevitable detours, acknowledge the fact that none of us are perfect. Stay optimistic. Turn your attention to health-promoting strategies. If your child is old enough, let her participate in this process of figuring out what went wrong and how you can prevent it from happening again.

So if grandma always brings a bag of candy whenever she visits, can you talk with her and suggest that she give her grandchildren nonfood gifts from now on? If you've backtracked from your commitment to cut back on trips to the local fried-chicken take-out restaurant, can you immediately do an about-face and return to healthier eating?

Once you reverse course and begin making positive changes, don't let down your guard and just assume that things will move forward without any further problems. Although some people think that they can make changes and then forget about them, you can't count on a smooth road ahead. You need to remain vigilant. Keep monitoring your child's progress in the weeks and months ahead. Make sure she doesn't fall back into old habits that could undermine all of her positive efforts to date.

Sneaking Food

It can happen at almost anytime. While you're talking on the phone, when you're taking a shower, when you're out running errands—without your knowledge and perhaps without you ever finding out, your overweight child may start sneaking food. When she's older, she may indulge at friends' homes, or when she has money, she may purchase her own treats.

Why is your youngster behaving this way? After all, she may truly want to lose weight, so why is she sneaking food behind your back? There are many possible explanations. Your child could be feeling anxiety over issues with friends, and she might find food soothing and comforting. She could be bored or tired. Or she may be sad or lonely. In many cases, she might interpret these emotions as hunger, and she'll raid the cupboard when no one's looking.

In most families, this sneaking of food doesn't go undetected for long. You might notice a few dirty dishes in her bedroom. Maybe there will be food items noticeably missing from the refrigerator. Perhaps you'll find candy wrappers in her waste basket.

In cases like these, what should you do?

First, don't panic or overreact. Raise the issue with your child. Without being accusatory and becoming angry or threatening to punish her, tell your child that you've noticed that she sometimes eats in her room when she thinks no one is looking. Explain that you're aware of her behavior. Point out that it's counterproductive to her weight-loss goals. Then agree to help your child work on the problem.

Some parents find it helpful to establish a rule that their children have to ask them (or their spouses) for food. Rather than simply telling your youngster, "Don't sneak!" encourage her to ask for food when she wants it. Explain that you'll help her make good nutritional decisions about what and when to eat. You can move her in the direction of sneaking less often and making better food choices when she does eat.

For example, you might say, "What kinds of foods have you been sneaking?"

Your child might respond, "I'm eating chips late at night."

You could follow up by asking, "Where do you get them?"

"I buy them from the vending machine at school."

"Well, when you feel like eating, can you make healthier decisions than reaching for chips? Next time you want some food, ask me. We'll choose foods together that can keep your weight-loss efforts moving in the right direction."

Once your child begins to ask you for food, reward her for doing so (although obviously don't reward her with food!). For a young child, give her a sticker or star each time she asks you for something to eat, or read her an extra bedtime story. She also can accumulate points for a low-cost toy or school supplies. For an older child, perhaps she can build up points for a ticket to the movies on Saturday afternoon or a day at the skating rink or zoo.

Snacking and Grazing and Your Child's Hunger

See if the following scenarios sound familiar:

- Your child sits down for dinner, but only nibbles at her meal, eating very little of it. Then 30 minutes after leaving the table, she comes into the kitchen, saying she's starving. Before you can utter a word, she starts gobbling up something from the refrigerator or cupboard, then returns to the scene of the crime again and again, grazing for food well into the night.
- Your child eats 3 highly structured, healthy meals a day that you carefully prepare, but then all those conscientious efforts toward good nutrition fall apart during her snacking, which at times seems as though it can turn into an all-day event.

For school-aged and adolescent kids, the biggest and most dangerous times for snacking are after school and after dinner. Typically, children will come home from school, and perhaps they're wound up, stressed out, or simply bored. So they reach for a pacifier in the form of food.

If your child seems to be overly reliant on snacking, take a look at what's going on. Use the questions in worksheet #14 on page 122 to help you better understand your child's snacking behavior, and then intervene.

As a general guideline, youngsters should consume 2 snacks a day—preferably low-calorie foods such as fruits and vegetables. Of course, if the decision making is left in their hands, many would opt for other types of snacks—potato chips, cookies, candy, French fries, or a slice of pizza or two. If it's high in fat and rich in calories, it seems to draw them like a magnet. How about steering your child toward snacks such as

- Carrots or celery sticks
- A cup of melon or strawberries
- Three cups of light microwave popcorn
- An apple
- A cup of vegetable soup
- Sugar-free gelatin or fruit snacks

You can add to this list of healthy snacks. These are the kinds of foods that will help your child end of the cycle of unhealthy eating.

At the same time, recommit yourself to making sure your child eats 3 well-balanced meals a day; that should help quench her appetite for anything more than 2 modest and healthy snacks. If she's snacking out of boredom or anxiety, one of your challenges is to help her deal with the emotions and life situations that are steering her toward food. Encourage your child to take part in this decision making. Ask her, "What can you do besides eat when you think you're hungry?" It sounds like a silly question, but some youngsters will give it some thought and then say, "Well, I can go outside," "I can play with my blocks," or, "I can read a book." Those options are a lot healthier than feeding his hunger, particularly when it really isn't hunger at all.

You may be surprised that she can give you some alternatives, or you may need to help her think of other things to do if she is stuck. Some ideas might be

- Walk the dog.
- Run through the sprinklers.
- Play a game of badminton.
- Kick a soccer ball.
- Paint a picture.
- Go in-line skating.
- Dance.
- Plant a flower in the garden.
- Fly a kite.
- Join you for a walk through the mall (without stopping at the ice cream shop).

Teasing and Bullying

Some obese children have to deal with more than just losing their excess weight. They are also teased at school, often unmercifully, because of their obesity. Over time, this taunting can take an emotional toll on any youngster, particularly as they lose friends and self-esteem. Some of these children eventually dread going to school at all. In fact,

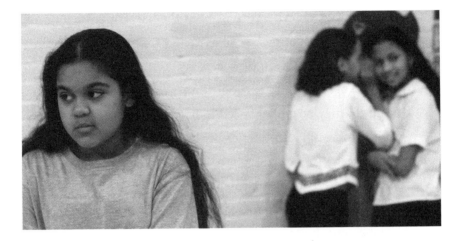

research shows that children who are bullied are more likely to skip going to class; some even drop out of school altogether.

In many cases, this taunting escalates with time. As it intensifies, these children may become terrified, even fearing for their physical safety. For parents, it can be heartbreaking to watch.

So how should you and your child respond to this bullying?

- Tell an adult.
- Stay in a group.
- As much as she possibly can, she should not react to the taunting. If the school bully sees her becoming anxious or even start to cry, the teasing is likely to get worse. Encourage your child to maintain her composure, turn around, and walk away.
- If the bullying continues, your child can, if she feels safe, try being assertive and stand up to her tormenter. In some cases, a firm statement will neutralize the confrontation—something like "Stop bugging me!" The bully might react by turning her attention to an "easier prey" who won't fight back and appears more vulnerable to verbal attacks.

- Let your child's teacher know about the harassment being directed at your youngster. The teacher may be able to intervene to put an end to it. If the teasing continues, ask the school principal or your child's school counselor to get involved. Your youngster may be embarrassed to have you talk to the principal, but you can't afford to let her be mistreated any further. In fact, many schools now have anti-bullying policies. It is generally better to let the teacher and principal handle the situation, rather than contacting the bully or the bully's parents yourself.

- Convince your child to try bonding more closely with the friends that she does have at school. If she hangs out with a group on the playground or in the lunch room, she is less likely to be singled out for mistreatment.

- Add an activity outside of school that your overweight child can participate in, during which she can develop a new peer group that may be less inclined to tease. Sign her up for a karate class or the Boy or Girl Scouts.

- Spend time with your child and treat her as an important person. Help maintain your child's self-esteem by demonstrating respect and acceptance and conveying the message, "I believe in you."

When you're evaluating the teasing to which your overweight child is subjected, don't overlook what may be going on in your own home. Sadly, some obese youngsters are teased by their own siblings. Even some parents direct negative comments at their overweight youngster, often with statements like, "I'm telling you what to do—why aren't you doing it?" If this is happening in your home, you need to put a stop to it. Have a family discussion about it, and set some sensible ground rules for relating to one another in a more positive way.

Child Care and School Issues

Because children spend so many hours a day in school or child care settings, one of your biggest parenting challenges is to stay up-to-date on what's going on there, including how it affects your child's health and well-being.

Of course, you should talk to your child daily about what's happening at school academically and socially. Who are her friends? Who does she eat lunch with? Where and what does she eat, in the school cafeteria and from vending machines? Does she share food with friends, perhaps exchanging the sack lunch you've prepared with a friend's lunch?

In a growing number of schools, children can use a school debit card to buy lunches and snacks, with parents adding monetary value to the card every week or month. If your child uses one of these cards, how closely are you keeping track of how she's spending the money? If those funds are disappearing too quickly, your child may be overeating and perhaps making poor nutritional choices. With regularity, you need to ask her, "What did you buy with the debit card today?" If you're not pleased with the answer, you may need to switch strategies. For example, begin giving your child lunch money every morning so she can't overspend on items that she'd be better off not eating.

As we pointed out earlier in the book, you need to use the same hands-on approach if your youngster attends a child care center. Do you know what she's eating there? How much physical activity is she getting?

If you think her nutrition at the child care facility isn't optimal, pack a lunch and a snack for your child each day. When preparing sandwiches, think healthy—turkey or lean roast beef rather than bologna or pastrami. Snacks may include yogurt, applesauce, pretzels, a piece of fruit, or low-fat string cheese. For drinks, choose bottled water or have your child buy a carton of low-fat milk.

Turn back to chapters 2 and 3 and review the suggestions made there for healthy eating and activity levels at school and child care. Remember to monitor what your child is eating. Even if you're having successes at home in improving her nutrition and activity level, the school environment can weaken those efforts if things are out of sync there.

When Time Becomes an Issue

Have you ever thought, "I know my child should be physically active, but there just aren't enough hours in the day. She's so busy with homework, clarinet lessons, and after-school clubs that she just doesn't have time to get outdoors and run around." Or, "We made the decision to cut down on how often we eat out, but we're always so pressed for time. By the time I leave work and pick up the kids at child care, there's just no time to cook. Our goal of once-a-week restaurant dining ends up being 3 or 4 times a week."

Refrains like these are common among today's parents. If you plan ahead, there are solutions to just about every problem as your child works at managing her weight. For example, it might be true that time is limited for meal preparation on weeknights, but you can simplify things and do some advance planning on the weekends. As you read in Chapter 2, dinners don't have to be elaborate. They can be as simple as a sandwich, bowl of soup, piece of fruit, and glass of milk. It's easier to do the right thing than you might think.

How about the sixth grader who complains that she can't play outside for even 15 minutes because "I have too much homework"? You need to sit down with her and plan in advance for those days when it seems impossible to find even 15 minutes for physical activity. Create a schedule to fit in the most important (and healthy) tasks and activities that should be part of her after-school hours. It may be that while she really does have plenty of homework, she might spend part of her homework time talking on the phone with a friend or answering e-mails on the computer. It may be easier than you think to find those extra 15 minutes, particularly when physical activity is a family priority.

Also, have a plan B ready when things don't unfold the way you thought they would. Even if you arrange your child's schedule carefully, have a fallback strategy when unforeseen circumstances arise. At the last minute, maybe your child's math teacher changes the midterm examination from Wednesday to Tuesday, and suddenly your youngster really will be studying well into the evening. Perhaps she has an orthodontist appointment that takes longer than you thought, and unexpectedly there's much less after-school time than you had anticipated. In cases like these, your plan B might include some indoor activity for your child after dark (maybe the family can exercise together to a workout video), and dinner might be a frozen entrée that you had prepared over the weekend and placed in the freezer. Rather than letting events overwhelm you and your child, think ahead about how you'll handle the unexpected.

Keep in mind that there's a difference between being busy and being active. A lot of today's children are very busy with after-school activities, including tutoring and music lessons. Being busy, however, doesn't necessarily translate into being physically active, which is something overweight children (and all children, for that matter) need. Kids must have balance in their lives, and exercise should be part of it. Activity needs to become a priority.

Vacations, Holidays, and Other Family Gatherings

Many children (as well as adults) tend to gain weight during holidays and vacations. On a weeklong trip to the beach, for example, families often let their nutrition and activity routines take a back seat to the events of the day. That's why it's helpful to think ahead and do some preparation before a vacation. Can the entire family agree to continue your healthy eating during your trip? Can you schedule some physical activity into your vacation, whether it's walking through the amusement park or swimming in the hotel pool? When you're on a trip, you shouldn't take a vacation from proper eating and exercise.

During holidays and other special occasions, don't lose sight of what your child is eating. Christmas and Hanukkah celebrations often last for much of December, with plenty of candy and cakes offering one temptation after another. In fact, for many families, the preoccupation with food extends from Thanksgiving through New Year's Day. No wonder you need to approach this time of year with extra care.

So how should you deal with the holidays? You certainly don't want to deprive your child of the celebrations. All of us, children and adults alike need these kinds of celebrations in our lives. But celebrate the day, not the entire month! Your child can enjoy the holiday, departing from her nutritional plan for just a day, and then go back to her plan for healthy eating.

The same is true for birthday parties, other religious holidays, and Halloween. If your child is invited to a friend's birthday party, she can certainly have some ice cream and cake. But remind her to take only one helping of the treat. On Easter Sunday, for example, she can have a little candy, but fill up most of her Easter basket with inexpensive toys, and don't make Easter a 2-week celebration overflowing with sugar-laden goodies. On Halloween, let your child trick or treat, but then suggest that she sell the candy to you for a negotiated amount. She'll get a few dollars, and you can dispose of the candy. Most children think that's a pretty good deal—besides, if the candy were to stay in the house instead, you just know someone would eat it! The key is to incorporate these occasions as parts of the family routine along with the family's day-to-day nutrition and activity patterns.

Now, what about other types of family gatherings? In some cultures, when extended families get together, it can turn into an absolute food feast, lasting from breakfast until the last light goes out after dark. Of course, extended families are important, but does your child really need to have huge helpings of food whenever you go over to her favorite uncle's house? In fact, it's important to think moderation when you're at relatives' homes. Family members— grandparents, aunts, and uncles—can have an enormous effect on your child's health. Invite them to support her in her journey toward better health. Let them know that you'd like them to become part of your child's health team.

Important Points to Remember

- Setbacks and backsliding should be viewed as minor stumbling blocks and not a reason to abandon all efforts for healthy change.
- Monitor your child's progress, and make certain she doesn't fall back into old habits with regularity.
- If your child is sneaking food, establish a rule that she has to ask you or your spouse for food.
- Children often snack not because they're hungry, but because they're bored, anxious, or tired.
- When it doesn't seem as if there are enough hours in the day, plan in advance and set priorities so you can fit what's most important into your family's schedule.
- During holidays, your child should celebrate with the family and not feel denied. Even so, limits need to be placed on the amount of sweets that are available.

WORKSHEET TO TAKE TO YOUR PEDIATRICIAN
#13: CONQUERING SETBACKS

Has your overweight child experienced a lapse in his or her progress toward better health? If a setback does take place, use this worksheet to help both of you understand and overcome the obstacles that may have tripped your child up. Remember, when trying to work through a setback, it's important to partner with your pediatrician.

What's Currently Happening?
What setback has occurred in your child's life that has interfered with his or her weight-loss efforts?

_____

_____

Did it happen just once, or repeatedly? _____ Is it still going on? _____

Why do you think this backsliding has occurred? Is there an event, a person, or a behavior that has contributed to the problem?

_____

_____

What Changes Need to Be Made and How Will You Make Them?
In the following space, write down a specific area in which a setback has occurred and where you and your child would like to make a change.

_____

_____

Are there obstacles that you and your youngster need to deal with effectively to ensure success in preventing this setback from recurring in the future?

_____

_____

What specific steps can you and your youngster take to make this change and minimize the risk of future setbacks?

_____

_____

Who can support you and your child in making these changes?

_____

WORKSHEET TO TAKE TO YOUR PEDIATRICIAN

#14: EVALUATING SNACKING BEHAVIORS

In this worksheet, we'll look at your child's snacking and ways in which problems can be effectively managed as the family navigates its way toward a healthier life.

What's Currently Happening With Snacking?
Are there certain times of day when your child snacks? _____

Does your child appear to snack because he or she is genuinely hungry? _____

Does your child make mostly healthy choices when he or she reaches for snacks?

_____

If so, what kinds of healthy snacks does your child choose?

_____

What Problems Exist With Snacking?
Does your child sometimes select snacks that provide poor nutrition? _____

If so, what kinds of snacks does your child tend to choose?

_____

Does your child's urge to snack, and do the snacking choices your child makes, seem to be affected by his or her mood or external events to which your child is reacting (for example, stressful situations, particular times of the day)?

_____

What Changes Need to Be Made and How Will You Make Them?
What obstacles are interfering with your child snacking on healthy foods and appropriate portion sizes?

_____

Select a problem area related to snacking with which your child is having difficulty (for example, snacking excessively when watching TV or doing homework). You and your child should create a specific plan for attacking this problem. Write down this approach here.

_____

_____

_____

Who can support you in making this change?

_____

7

Before and After Your Baby Is Born:
The Prenatal and Neonatal Periods

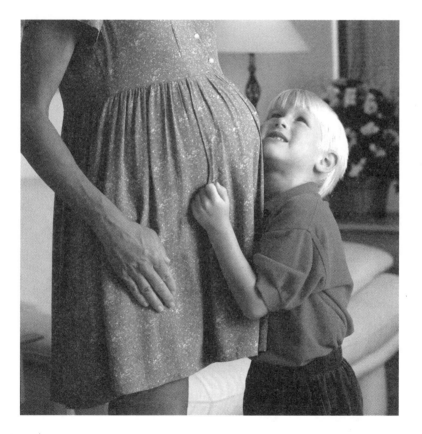

In this chapter and those that follow, we'll concentrate on specific developmental periods in your child's life. We'll examine the issues most relevant to these times of life that may contribute to your youngster's risk of becoming obese. Remember that it is always a good time to focus on improving your child's nutrition and activity, so if you have a child who has come into your life through adoption or foster care, you can start right where you are to make healthy nutrition and activity choices for your new arrival.

We'll begin here by concentrating on issues to consider if you are pregnant. Although you want your child to avoid becoming obese throughout his life, your primary focus during this prenatal period is to ensure that mom stays as healthy as possible during the 9 months of pregnancy, which in turn will help ensure good health for the baby.

Good nutrition starts in the womb and during your pregnancy. You should work closely with your obstetrician and later with your pediatrician, following their advice to make certain that your baby thrives in the womb and the immediate weeks and months after birth. Your goal should be to get the best possible, complete prenatal care, including attention to what you should be eating, your weight gain, and the physical activity you should be getting.

If you don't yet have a pediatrician, use the time during your pregnancy to select one and begin developing a relationship with him or her (see "Selecting a Pediatrician" on page 131). If you and/or your spouse are overweight or if other close relatives are obese, talk to your pediatrician about your baby's risk of developing a weight problem and how you can reduce that risk. Believe it or not, a genetic tendency to obesity, especially an overweight mother, is a strong factor influencing your child's risk of obesity.

Optimizing Your Own Nutrition

Throughout your pregnancy, you'll be eating not only for yourself, but for your baby, as well (it's really true that you should be "eating for 2" when you're pregnant). With the guidance of your obstetrician, you need to *increase* the amount of calories, protein, and minerals you consume. If you have an overweight problem yourself and have been a constant dieter who latches onto one fad diet after another, your pregnancy is a time to set aside those diets and eat more healthfully, for your baby's sake.

Bear in mind that for your newborn, good nutrition starts in the womb. Your obstetrician will advise you to eat sensible, well-balanced meals that include extra calories, protein, minerals, and other nutrients to keep your baby growing normally in the uterus. Remember, these nutrients will make their way to your growing baby, so be thoughtful about what you choose to put on your plate, making sure you consume a variety of foods from all food groups.

If your obstetrician recommends prenatal vitamin tablets, take them as suggested, but don't self-prescribe any other supplements until you discuss them with your doctor. You should also stay away from all medications, including over-the-counter pills, except those specifically recommended by your obstetrician. Many mothers have questions about taking certain medications (for example, cold or allergy medications) during pregnancy. This is normal; your obstetrician can answer these questions for you during prenatal visits.

This is also a good time to begin planning your newborn's nutrition for the first months and years of life. Refer back to Chapter 2, and start thinking about how you can nourish your child in ways that keep him healthy without increasing his risk of obesity.

Are You Going to Breastfeed?

Most mothers decide how they wish to feed their new babies long before they deliver. So while you are pregnant, you need to decide whether you're going to breastfeed your new baby or feed him formula. The American Academy of Pediatrics (AAP) strongly advocates the use of breastfeeding exclusively for approximately the first 6 months of your baby's life, which is about the age at which you'll start to add solid foods to his diet (see "Where the American Academy of Pediatrics Stands" on page 129). You shouldn't feel guilty if you cannot breastfeed or decide to feed your baby formula instead—it can provide an adequate balance of fat, protein, and sugar that your baby requires. However, with formula feeding, there is a higher risk of your baby developing ear infections, episodes of vomiting and diarrhea, and upper respiratory infections during the first year of life.

There are many good reasons to breastfeed. You should know that breastfeeding and/or breast milk

- Provides all of the nutritional requirements that your newborn needs in the initial months of life to grow and develop normally.
- Gives your baby antibodies to help protect him against germs like bacteria and viruses, including those that cause ear infections, diarrhea, vomiting, urinary tract infections, pneumonia, and even bacterial meningitis. Breastfed babies also have a lower incidence of diabetes, asthma, and other chronic diseases.
- Offers protection against crib death or sudden infant death syndrome.
- Allows mother and baby to bond emotionally during feeding in a special way. Breastfeeding encourages skin-to-skin contact between mother and baby, as well as time for cuddling with and comforting your baby.
- Is economical and, most mothers believe, more convenient— it requires no preparation (such as heating up a bottle) before each feeding.
- Is healthy for mothers as well, significantly reducing their risk of breast and ovarian cancer, as well as making them less susceptible to hip fractures and osteoporosis later in life.

Next, what about your baby's likelihood of becoming overweight? Can breastfeeding lower this risk? More research is needed to definitively answer these questions. But studies thus far show that breastfeeding probably is an important factor in reducing the prevalence of child obesity. No, it won't completely eliminate your youngster's chances of becoming overweight, but it does appear to have a definite effect on lowering the risk. In one recent study published in the AAP journal *Pediatrics,* the rate of being overweight was highest among children who were never breastfed or were breastfed for less than 1 month. Another study concluded that at 1 year of age, breastfed babies are leaner than formula-fed babies.

In your initial meeting or two with your baby's pediatrician, talk with the doctor about whether breastfeeding makes the most sense for you and your baby. Keep in mind that if you're unsure of the method you will use to feed your baby, you can always begin breastfeeding, see how it goes, and decide later if or when to add formula.

Where the American Academy of Pediatrics Stands

In our most recent (2005) policy statement about breastfeeding, the American Academy of Pediatrics confirmed its strong advocacy of exclusively breastfeeding babies for approximately the first 6 months* of life. We also support continued breastfeeding for the entire first year of life and beyond, as long as that is desired by mother and baby.

If you are breastfeeding your baby, the policy statement also recommends having your pediatrician (or another experienced health care professional) evaluate your newborn when he is 3 to 5 days old (usually 1 or 2 days after discharge home from the hospital) and again at 2 to 3 weeks of age, to be certain that he is feeding and growing normally. This early checkup right after discharge is most important to make sure that your breastfeeding is coming along normally.

*There is a difference of opinion among American Academy of Pediatrics experts on this matter. The Section on Breastfeeding supports exclusive breastfeeding for about 6 months. The Committee on Nutrition supports the introduction of complementary foods between 4 and 6 months of age where safe and nutritious complementary foods are available.

If you choose to start with formula feeding right after birth, it can be very difficult to switch to breastfeeding further down the road.

Your pediatrician may be able to recommend a lactation consultant or a class in breastfeeding to help you get started in breastfeeding. Lactation consultants are often nurses or dietitians with special training in teaching the fundamentals of breastfeeding and managing breastfeeding problems. Some of these consultants will come to your home after your baby is born if you're having difficulties. They will work with your pediatrician to help you successfully breastfeed your baby and see that your baby is growing normally.

Are You Physically Active?

Despite all the changes that are taking place in your body during pregnancy, this is no time to abandon your own efforts to stay physically active. Most women can exercise throughout their pregnancies, following the advice of their obstetricians on the types of physical activity that are most appropriate for them. You might decide to take regular walks through your neighborhood, swim at the YMCA or in your backyard pool, garden, or play golf. In general, most mild to moderate forms of exercise are healthy for you and your developing baby. However, your doctor will probably discourage activities that involve jumping or jolting movements, like running or jumping rope.

If you have certain pregnancy-related health conditions, your obstetrician might suggest avoiding exercise altogether. If you have high blood pressure related to your pregnancy, persistent bleeding, or a high risk of preterm labor, for example, be sure to talk with your doctor before exercising.

Selecting a Pediatrician

Choosing a pediatrician is an important decision that you should make before your baby is born. Once your newborn arrives, it will be comforting to know that you have a pediatrician available who can care for your baby from birth, give him his very first examination, and answer all of your questions.

New parents sometimes interview several pediatricians before making their choices. These interviews can usually be arranged during the last few months of your pregnancy. If you need the names of a few pediatricians, you can ask your obstetrician and check with the American Academy of Pediatrics Web site under the section "Find a Pediatrician." You can also ask friends and family members with children about the pediatricians they use and whether they're happy with their choices. You want to select a pediatrician that you feel you can talk to.

During your interviews with these pediatricians, ask them questions like, "How soon after birth will you see my baby for his first examination?" "At what intervals do you recommend seeing newborns for healthy baby visits?" "Are you willing to respond to questions by telephone?" "When you're unavailable, what pediatrician will I be able to reach instead?" "What procedures do you advise following in case of an emergency?" and "What are the fees for the health care services you provide, and do you accept the insurance my family has?"

Many additional topics discussed in this chapter and throughout the book can be raised during your interviews and subsequent visits to the pediatrician's office, including the benefits of breastfeeding and the prevention and management of obesity in children.

Important Points to Remember

- The prenatal period is an important time to help ensure the good health of your baby.

- Good nutrition starts in the womb. Be thoughtful about what you choose to eat.

- Because you'll be eating for 2, you'll need to increase your intake of calories, protein, and minerals, while following the advice of your physician.

- The AAP recommends exclusive breastfeeding for approximately the first 6 months of your baby's life (see "Where the American Academy of Pediatrics Stands" on page 129).

- Breastfeeding your baby may help to reduce his risk of becoming overweight.

- Maintain an active lifestyle throughout your pregnancy with the guidance of your doctor.

WORKSHEET TO TAKE TO YOUR PEDIATRICIAN

#15: YOUR FAMILY'S WELL-BEING: PAST, PRESENT, AND FUTURE

In this worksheet, let's look at some of the issues that are particularly relevant as you and your family prepare for a new addition to your household. You and your spouse should answer these questions and use the information as a starting point for conversation and possible change.

Are you and/or your spouse currently overweight? _____

Have you had a weight problem in the past? _____

What was your pre-pregnancy weight? _____

What was the pre-pregnancy weight of the baby's other biological parent? _____

Were you ever told you had pregnancy-related diabetes or gestational diabetes, or were you given a medicine to help control your blood sugar during pregnancy? _____

Have you previously had a very large baby (for example, 9 pounds or greater weight at birth)? _____

If you have other children, has obesity been a problem in their lives? _____

Use the following space to describe your own nutritional habits. For example, do you and your spouse eat balanced meals that can contribute to good health and normal weight? Or do you overrely on high-fat foods at the expense of healthier choices like fruits and vegetables? Elaborate.

_____

_____

_____

If you have other children, are they eating mostly nutritious meals? _____

What are typical breakfasts, lunches, and dinners like for your family these days?

_____

_____

In a typical week, how many times does your family eat at fast-food restaurants?

_____

If you've tried to cut back, how successful have you been?

_____

(Worksheet continues on page 134)

Are there nutritional areas in which you'd like your family to improve?

_____

_____

Are you physically active most days? _____

What forms of exercise do you enjoy participating in? _____

If you have other children, what kind of physical activity do they get at school and home and with what regularity?

_____

_____

How much television do your children currently watch per day?

_____

How often and when do you use the TV as a babysitter?

_____

What can you do in the present and future to make sure that your children participate in more physical activity?

_____

_____

What else can you do differently to create an environment for your new child that is compatible with avoiding or overcoming problems with overweight?

_____

_____

_____

_____

WORKSHEET TO TAKE TO YOUR PEDIATRICIAN

#16: TOPICS TO DISCUSS WITH YOUR PEDIATRICIAN

Before your next appointment with your baby's pediatrician, take a few moments to fill in the following information and then make a list of questions you want to ask the doctor. Tell your pediatrician that you'd like to look at your child's growth chart during every office visit so you can follow his or her progress.

What Is Currently Happening With Your Baby?
How is your baby's overall health? _____

Are you breastfeeding or formula feeding your baby? _____

Does your baby seem to be eating normally? _____

How often is your baby breastfeeding? _____

Does your baby seem satisfied after nursing? _____

Do you feel that you have to supplement your breastfeeding with formula? _____

How much formula does your baby take at each feeding? _____

Do your baby's motor skills appear to be developing normally, particularly when compared to other children the same age? _____

Does your baby watch TV? _____

If so, how many hours does your baby watch in a typical day? (Remember, TV is not recommended for children younger than 2 years.) _____

What Is Going Well?
Use the answers to the previous questions to help you determine and write down areas in which your baby is already being successful in the journey toward good health.

_____

_____

What Problems Exist With Your Baby?
Are there health issues in your baby's life that concern you? _____

If you've chosen to breastfeed, are you having any difficulties doing so? _____

Do you have any concerns about your baby's appetite? _____

Do you always or usually react to your baby's cries by feeding him or her?

Do you use a pacifier with your baby? _____

If you've started your baby on solid foods, are there any feeding problems that you've encountered?

_____

(Worksheet continues on page 136)

Are there other nutrition-related issues that concern you?

_____

_____

What Changes Do You Need to Make and How Can You Make Them?
What obstacles are preventing you from making changes to resolve the problems
you've identified?

_____

_____

With your pediatrician's help, identify ways in which you can resolve these
problems, step by step. Begin by singling out one problem and determining
(and listing) ways in which you can start attacking this concern. Next, work
to turn the problem into a success.

_____

_____

_____

Use the following space to note any additional issues or questions that you'd
like to discuss with your pediatrician about your baby's nutrition, physical
activity, and other issues relevant to keeping your baby healthy. Take this
list with you to your pediatrician's office.

_____

_____

_____

_____

8

The First Year

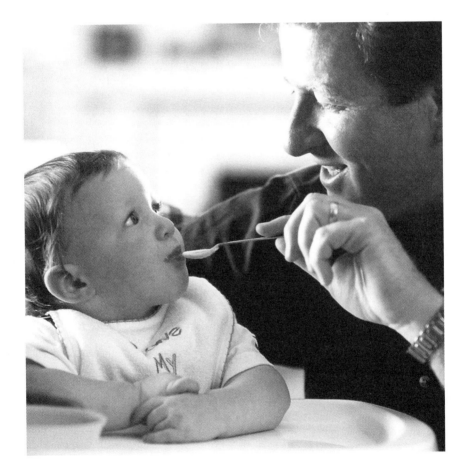

There are few life experiences more exciting than welcoming a new baby into the family. Even though it's such an exhilarating and enjoyable time for you and your spouse, there are probably some moments when you simply feel overwhelmed. You might ask yourself questions like, "Am I doing everything right to get my baby off to a good start?" "Am I giving her all the nourishment she needs?" "What else should I be doing to make sure she stays on the path toward good health?"

Particularly if you as parents struggle with weight problems or have an older child who's overweight, you might already be focused on how to prevent your new baby from developing a weight problem in childhood. Keep in mind, however, that your primary concern in this first year of your baby's life is not her weight, it's her overall health.

When your baby was born, her birth weight was influenced by a number of factors. Was she a full-term baby, or born prematurely? Were there any complications during your pregnancy (for example, if mom's blood pressure was high while pregnant, the baby might be a little small)? Did mom consume a well-balanced diet during the 9-month pregnancy, or was her own nourishment deficient? Did you get good and regular prenatal care?

Now that your baby has been born and is probably occupying many or most of your waking hours, your attention should be on her good health. Of course, during this first year of life, you'll notice the normal baby fat that all babies have. Most babies appear a little chubby. Don't overreact. Don't let your eyes deceive you. Parents and grandparents have all kinds of ideas of what babies should look like and how much weight they should be gaining. Trust your pediatrician to monitor your baby on a growth chart and let you know if she is growing normally.

Feeding Your Baby: Breast or Bottle?

In Chapter 7, you read about the benefits of breastfeeding. Good nutrition is essential at all ages of childhood, beginning at birth, and as we've emphasized, human milk is the best possible food for babies. That's why the American Academy of Pediatrics (AAP) recommends that you exclusively breastfeed your baby for about the first 6 months of life (see "Where the American Academy of Pediatrics Stands" on page 129). We also support continued breastfeeding for the entire first year and beyond, as long as mother and baby desire it.

But what if you've chosen to feed your baby with formula instead? To repeat the message in Chapter 7, don't feel guilty. Your baby will do all right being nourished with formula. Formula is a good source of nutrition, providing a healthy balance of fat, protein, and sugar, as well as plenty of vitamins and minerals such as iron, calcium, and vitamins C, D, and K. When consuming formula, your baby will have all her nutritional needs met so she can grow into a healthy child and adult.

Even so, breastfeeding is still our first choice, and it's something that you should strongly consider.

How Often and How Much Should Your Baby Eat?

Breastfed babies generally eat more frequently than those who are formula fed. Newborns usually nurse on their mothers' breasts every 2 to 3 hours; as they become older, the time between feedings will increase as the capacity of their stomachs becomes larger. By contrast, formula-fed newborns will start out by eating approximately every 3 to 4 hours during the first few weeks of life.

When you hold your baby to feed her a bottle, watch for cues that she is full, instead of using the clock as a guide. It's more important that you are attentive to clues or signals from your baby that indicate she's hungry. These are called *hunger cues.* When she wants to eat, she may become more alert, put her hands or fingers on or in her mouth, make sucking motions, stick out her tongue, smack her lips, kick or squirm, or begin *rooting* (moving her jaw and mouth or head in search of your breast). If she begins crying, this is usually a late signal that she wants to eat.

Whether breastfeeding or formula feeding, most parents worry about whether their babies are getting enough to eat. Because babies suck not only for hunger, but also for comfort, this can be hard to know at first. Even when babies no longer act hungry, some parents worry about whether all of their nutritional needs are being met.

Again, don't panic. Your baby will let you know when she's had enough or wants more. In most cases, she'll consume about 90% of the available breast milk during the first 10 minutes of feeding on each breast. Then she might move away from the breast or simply doze off. Among the many advantages of breastfeeding is that it tends to be cued or on-demand feeding, meaning that in a sense, your baby will take charge of her own feedings. If you watch your baby's responses, you should be able to figure out when she's full. She may turn her head or give other signals that she's no longer interested in eating. The formula-fed baby will also let you know when she's had enough. You might notice her becoming distracted while drinking from the bottle, or she might start fidgeting or turn her head. She may close her mouth tightly. As your baby gets a little older and her eye-to-hand coordination gets better, she might try to knock the bottle or spoon out of your grip.

On the other hand, if your baby finishes a bottle and starts smacking her lips or begins to cry, she probably wants more. On average, by the end of the first month, she should be taking in at least 4 ounces of formula per feeding. At 6 months of age, she'll be consuming 6 to 8 ounces per feeding.

You can also rely on your baby's diapers to give you clues on whether she's getting enough to eat. In the first month of your newborn's life, she should wet her diaper 6 or more times a day and have 3 to 4 (often more) bowel movements each day. Your baby should also appear satisfied for a couple of hours after each feeding if she's consuming adequate amounts of food.

What if your baby almost always seems to be hungry—or what if she doesn't appear to have the appetite that you think she should? If that's the case, talk to your pediatrician. The doctor will be able to answer specific questions or respond to your concerns about whether your baby is getting enough nourishment and is growing normally. During each office visit, the pediatrician is already keeping track of your baby's weight gain and monitoring whether her weight is continuing to increase steadily. For instance,

- From months 1 through 4 of life, your baby should gain about $1\frac{1}{2}$ to 2 pounds each month, while growing about 1 to $1\frac{1}{2}$ inches.
- Between 4 and 7 months of age, she'll add another 1 to $1\frac{1}{2}$ pounds per month and grow about 2 to 3 inches in length.
- By 8 months, the average boy will weigh between $14\frac{1}{2}$ and $17\frac{1}{2}$ pounds, while girls will probably weigh about a half-pound less.
- At 1 year of age, the typical child weighs about 3 times her birth weight.
- Breastfed babies tend to be chubbier than formula-fed babies during the first 4 to 6 months of life. Then they usually become leaner than formula-fed babies by 9 months to 1 year of age.

For more information about breastfeeding, we recommend the AAP book, *New Mother's Guide to Breastfeeding.*

A Crying Baby: What Does It Mean?

When your baby cries, how do you react? Many parents instinctively think that's she's hungry and needs to be fed. But there could be other reasons for her tears. Rather than immediately feeding your baby, take a moment to assess whether something else might be going on. Is she crying because she's uncomfortable, wet, or soiled? Is she sleepy? Is she having gas pains? Is she annoyed and irritated by noise and other stimuli that she finds too intense? Or is she ill (have you checked to see if she has a fever, for example)?

With time, you'll find yourself becoming much better at differentiating among your baby's cries. You'll know when she's really hungry or whether she just wants to be held or needs her diaper changed. Hunger cries tend to be short and low-pitched and rise and fall. A cry of distress or pain starts suddenly, is particularly loud, and tends to be a high-pitched shriek followed by a lengthy pause and then a flat wail.

No matter what the reason for your baby's tears, you should always respond to her needs. If you've just fed her, she's probably not hungry, and if nothing else seems to be awry, try letting her nurse some more or suck on a pacifier. Try rocking your baby or singing or talking to her. Gently stroke her head. Wrap her snugly in a receiving blanket, or walk with her in your arms or a stroller. The more time babies spend being held by their mothers, the less they cry. Remember, you cannot spoil a newborn baby.

Getting Started With Solid Foods

When your infant is able to sit independently and grab for things to put in her mouth, it's time to begin introducing solid foods. Start with simple, basic foods such as rice cereal. You should add breast milk or warm formula to the cereal, mixing about 1 tablespoon of cereal with every 4 to 5 tablespoons of breast milk. Look for infant cereals that are fortified with iron, which can provide about 30% to 45% of your infant's daily iron needs. About midway through the first year, her natural stores of iron will have become depleted, so extra iron is a good idea.

Here are some additional recommendations to keep in mind.

- Introduce your baby to other solid foods gradually. Good initial choices are other simple cereals, such as oatmeal, as well as vegetables and fruits. Most pediatricians recommend offering vegetables before offering fruits.

- Start these new foods one at a time, at intervals of every 2 to 3 days. This approach will allow your infant to become used to the taste and texture of each new food. It can also help you identify any food sensitivities or allergies that may develop as each new food is started. Some pediatricians advise introducing wheat and mixed cereals last because young babies could have allergic reactions to them. Contact your doctor if symptoms (for example, diarrhea, vomiting, rash) develop that seem to be related to particular foods.

- In the beginning, feed your infant small serving sizes—even just 1 to 2 small spoonfuls to start.

- Within about 2 to 3 months after starting solid foods, your infant should be consuming a daily diet that includes not only breast milk or formula, but also cereal, vegetables, fruits, and meats, divided among 3 meals.

- When your infant is about 8 to 9 months old, give her *finger* foods or table foods that she can pick up and feed to herself. Make sure she's not putting anything into her mouth that's large enough to cause choking. Do not give small infants raisins, nuts, popcorn, or small or hard food pieces that can be easily aspirated.

Low Fat? Low Calories?

If you're concerned about your child becoming obese, you might be tempted to feed her only low-fat solid foods to help keep her weight at normal levels. Here's a very important recommendation to keep in mind—*do not restrict your child's consumption of dietary fat and calories in the first 2 years of life.* In other words, don't put a baby younger than 2 years on a diet or give her low-fat or skim milk.

Here's why: the early months and years of your child's life are critical for the normal development of her brain and body. Specifically, she'll need calories from dietary fat for her brain to grow and mature normally. As a general rule, your child should get about half of her daily calories from fat up to the age of 2 years. After that, you can reduce those fat calories gradually; by 4 to 5 years, fat calories should provide about one third of your youngster's daily calories. Many families can be transitioned from whole cow's milk to skim or fat-free milk by gradually changing from whole milk to 2%, then to 1%, and then to skim milk. Some mothers even mix these together to make the changes imperceptible to their children.

Whether you've decided to breastfeed or formula feed your baby, either choice should provide your baby with all the fat she needs. However, when preparing formula, be sure to follow the label instructions carefully, adding the recommended amount of water. Formula is designed to provide about 20 calories per ounce, including the proper amount of fat to ensure optimal growth. If you weaken or dilute the formula by adding too much water, you can interfere with your baby's normal physical growth and brain development.

A Typical Menu for Your 8- to 12-Month-Old

Do you need some information and support in preparing a day's worth of meals for your infant? Your pediatrician is the best source of this kind of guidance, but here is a sample menu of the daily food consumption for an infant 8 to 12 months old. Use it to help you choose not only the types of foods for your infant, but also the appropriate serving sizes.

Breakfast

- One-fourth to $^1/_2$ cup of cereal or mashed egg yolk
- One-fourth to $^1/_2$ cup of fruit (diced)
- Four to 6 oz of breast milk/formula (4 oz = $^1/_2$ cup)

Snack

- Four to 6 oz of breast milk/formula
- One-fourth cup of cheese (diced) or cooked vegetables

Lunch

- One-fourth to $^1/_2$ cup of yogurt or cottage cheese
- One-fourth to $^1/_2$ cup of yellow vegetables
- Four to 6 oz of breast milk/formula

Snack

- One teething biscuit or cracker
- One-fourth cup of cheese (diced) or meat

Dinner

- One-fourth cup of poultry, meat, or tofu (diced)
- One-fourth to $^1/_2$ cup of green vegetables
- One-fourth cup of rice or potato
- One-fourth cup of fruit
- Four to 6 oz of breast milk/formula

Before Bedtime

- Six to 8 oz of breast milk/formula or water

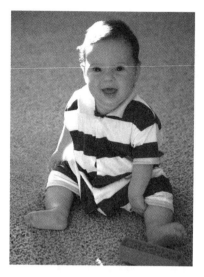

How Active Is Your Baby?

You might not think of the first few weeks of your baby's life as being a time when she's very physically active (although you will probably feel that you and your spouse are being run ragged in caring for her!). True, she's certainly not able to run through the park or throw a ball to another child at this age, but there are still many opportunities for her to begin to develop motor skills that she can build on for a very active childhood and adult life.

For example, have you noticed that your infant has started kicking during the second month of life? Even though this movement is mostly reflective at this point, before long she'll be able to flex and straighten her legs whenever she wants to. By the time she's 3 months old, your infant may be able to start kicking herself over from her front to her back (later, by 6 months of age, she'll start rolling from back to front). At about 3 to 4 months, when you hold her upright with her feet resting on the floor, she'll push down and straighten her legs as though she were standing on her own, and she'll probably discover that she can bend her knees and bounce.

Beginning at about 5 months of age, your infant will be able to raise her head while lying on her stomach and then push up on her arms to lift her chest off the floor or bed. Rocking on her tummy, she may kick her legs and move her arms as though she were swimming.

Before long, your infant will be rolling over at will. At about 8 months, she'll be able to sit without support and catch herself with her arms and hands if she starts to topple over. She'll also pick up and move objects from one hand to the other.

In the last few months before her first birthday, your infant may seem like she's in constant motion. She'll grab her feet and try putting them in her mouth. She may fidget and kick throughout every diaper change. Between 7 and 10 months of age, she'll begin experimenting with and then mastering the art of crawling. Next, right around the time of her first birthday, she'll take her first steps (it may happen a little earlier or a little later from one child to the next, all within a normal range).

As your baby develops, take advantage of every opportunity to help stimulate her mind and body. From the earliest weeks of life, walk around the house while holding and interacting with your baby and say aloud the names of the objects that the 2 of you encounter. Before long, she'll want to reach out, touch them, and pick them up. Also, talk to your baby whenever you're with her. Whether you're changing her diaper, bathing her, or driving with her in the car, keep the conversation going. Babies love the sound of their parents' voices. See how she responds and how she communicates with sounds by moving her arms and legs.

Here are some other activities that you and your baby can do together.

- Read out loud to your baby.
- Play some music and gently dance with her in your arms.
- Sit and play with her on the floor. She will love interacting with you.

- Try teaching her peekaboo and patty-cake (they can be stimulating for your baby and will help her develop motor skills).
- Hug her frequently and provide her with loving physical contact.
- Hold your baby as often as you can.
- Put her in the stroller and take her for a walk. It's a good way to expose your child to the world around her, and it's great exercise for you.

As your baby continues to grow and develop, her level of activity will increase. Make sure she has safe and soft toys to play with. They should be small enough so she can pick them up, but large enough so she can't put them in her mouth.

Television Watching and Young Children

Some parents mistakenly think that watching television is one way for babies to develop their understanding of words and language and identify human faces. Instead, babies love looking at and listening to moms' or dads' faces and interact with siblings or other caregivers.

Placing babies in bouncy seats in front of TVs might seem like a great way for them to exercise and perhaps a chance for moms and dads to rest for a few minutes. But TV isn't appropriate for children younger than 2 years. It only takes time away from meaningful interactions that your baby could be having with you and other family members.

As we've already emphasized in this book, TV watching is not a health-promoting activity for children. In fact, excessive TV watching is associated with obesity and overweight in children. You should be looking for opportunities to relate to and communicate with your child, rather than using the TV set as a babysitter. That's why the AAP has taken a strong stand against TV watching for very young children in particular.

Where the American Academy of Pediatrics Stands

In the first 2 years of life, your child's brain and body are going through very critical periods of growth and development. During this time, it is important for your youngster to have positive interactions with other people, including adults and children, and not sit idly in front of the TV.

For that reason, the American Academy of Pediatrics currently recommends that TV should not be watched by children 2 years and younger. For older children, TV watching (of educational, nonviolent programming) should be limited to no more than 1 to 2 hours a day.

WORKSHEET TO TAKE TO YOUR PEDIATRICIAN
#17: THE FIRST YEAR

Before your next appointment with your baby's pediatrician, take a few moments to fill in the following information and make a list of questions you want to ask the doctor. Tell your pediatrician that you'd like to look at your child's growth chart during every office visit so you can follow your child's progress.

What Is Currently Happening With Your Baby?
How is your baby's overall health? _____

Are you breastfeeding or formula feeding your baby? _____

Does your baby seem to be eating normally? _____

Do your baby's motor skills appear to be developing normally, particularly when compared to other babies the same age? _____

Do you sit your baby in front of the TV? _____

What activities do you participate in with your baby to encourage motor and mental development?

_____

_____

What Is Going Well?
Use the answers to the previous questions to help you determine and write down those areas in which your baby is already being successful in the journey toward good health.

_____

_____

_____

What Problems Exist With Your Baby?
Are there health issues in your baby's life that concern you?

_____

_____

If you've chosen to breastfeed, are you having any difficulties doing so?

_____

Do you have any concerns about your baby's appetite? _____

Do you always or usually react to your baby's cries by feeding him or her? _____

If you've started your infant on solid foods, are there any feeding problems that you've encountered?

_____

_____

Are there other nutrition-related issues that concern you?

_____

What Changes Do You Need to Make and How Can You Make Them?
What obstacles are preventing you from making changes to resolve the problems you've identified?

_____

_____

With your pediatrician's help, identify ways in which you can resolve these problems, step by step. Begin by singling out one problem, then determine and list ways in which you can start attacking this concern. Next, work to turn the problem into a success.

_____

_____

Use the following space to note any additional issues or questions that you'd like to discuss with your pediatrician about your baby's nutrition, physical activity, and other issues relevant to keeping him or her healthy. Take this list with you to your pediatrician's office.

_____

_____

_____

_____

9

The Toddler Years

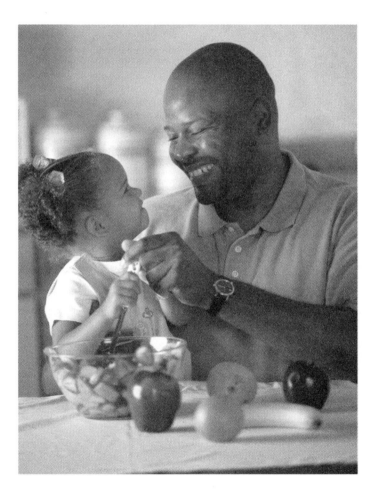

*A*s your baby has become a toddler, this can be a particularly pleasurable—and challenging—time for you as a parent. Although he's speaking in only 1- or 2-word sentences, he has enough language skills to communicate whether and when he's hungry and even verbally express his preferences about the particular foods he wants. At this stage in life, your toddler can feed himself with his hands, although he's also learning to use a spoon and drink from a cup. His food preferences may change frequently, and his appetite can increase or decrease from day to day, seemingly on a whim.

This is also a time when, after his first birthday, your toddler's growth rate actually starts to slow, which is quite normal. Yes, his height and weight will increase steadily, but not as rapidly as it did in the first months of life. In his entire second year, he'll gain an average of 3 to 5 pounds. So, for example,

- When your daughter is 15 months old, she'll weigh (on average) about 22 pounds and measure nearly 31 inches tall. Over the next 3 months, she'll gain about $1\frac{1}{2}$ pounds and grow about an inch. By her second birthday, she'll weigh about 27 pounds and measure about 34 inches.
- When your son is 15 months old, he'll weigh an average of about 24 pounds, and measure 31 inches. Over the next 3 months, he'll gain an average of $1\frac{1}{2}$ pounds and grow an additional inch. By the time of his second birthday, he'll weigh nearly 28 pounds and measure 36 inches.

These numbers will give you a general sense of the typical growth rates of toddlers. However, keep this important point in mind—children of the same age can vary significantly in their sizes and rates of growth and still fall within the normal range. Despite these wide variations, some parents are already becoming worried that their toddlers are overweight. They might express those concerns to their pediatricians. Even more troubling, they might decide on their own to put their toddlers on diets, which can unwittingly reduce the youngsters' intake of the essential nutrients they need for normal growth. There are risks when parents overreact by altering their children's diets in unhealthy ways.

Rely on Your Pediatrician

In a society that seems to revere thinness while simultaneously dealing with a growing epidemic of obesity, it's not surprising that your child's weight gets some of your attention. At this time in your child's life, don't let yourself become preoccupied with what he weighs. Every time you and your youngster visit the pediatrician's office, the doctor will track your child's height and weight on a growth chart, which is the most reliable way to gauge whether he falls outside the normal range.

Your pediatrician should be able to ease any anxieties you have. The doctor may explain that as babies evolve into toddlers, their muscles develop, they'll become more active, and they'll begin to lose some of the baby fat that may have given them a chubby appearance. In fact, a toddler's percentage of body fat will tend to gradually decrease as he continues to get older.

However, your pediatrician won't rely solely on visual observation to determine whether your child's weight is just right. The most reliable guide is where your child's height and weight fall on a standard growth chart. If the chart shows that your toddler is a little heavier than normal, your pediatrician can determine what actions, if any, are most appropriate at this age. As a general rule, however, you should never restrict calories in a toddler (up to the age of 3 years) without the guidance of your pediatrician because you don't want to risk interfering with his normal growth and development.

For most children, the proper health-promoting strategies are quite uncomplicated. They involve guidance that you've heard before.

- Optimize your child's nutrition.
- Make sure he gets plenty of physical activity.

Optimizing Nutrition

Since his very first feeding, you've probably paid plenty of attention to what your child eats. Remember, in making dietary decisions early in your youngster's life, your primary focus should be on good nutrition rather than the number of calories he's consuming. Instead of trying to limit the amount of dietary fat on your toddler's plate, introduce him to healthy eating habits and well-balanced meals and snacks, rather than approaches aimed specifically at losing weight.

So what should your toddler be eating? At 1 year of age, he should be consuming a wide variety of foods. As he moves through the second year of life, he should be eating 3 meals daily, along with 1 to 2 snacks, prepared and served at regular times. You should also discourage grazing (this means your child has access to and grabs food all day long).

In planning and preparing food for your toddler, make sure he's getting a balance of fats, protein, carbohydrates, vitamins, and minerals that can promote growth and include foods from the major food groups each day, including

- Meat, poultry, fish, eggs
- Dairy products such as milk and cheese
- Cereal grains, rice, potatoes, breads, pasta
- Vegetables and fruits

By choosing health-promoting foods, you can establish good nutritional habits in your child that will last for the rest of his life. However, one recent study found that about 65% to 70% of 1- to 2-year-olds ate dessert, ice cream, and/or candy once a day, and 30% to 50% drank sweetened beverages every day. By contrast, the same study indicated that less than 10% of these young children ate a dark green vegetable each day; more often, their vegetable intake consisted of potatoes and french fries. Make sure that you and the other adults in the family agree on a healthy nutritional lifestyle for your toddler and the entire family, including one that puts a limit on sweets.

For help in making good food choices, review the dietary recommendations in Chapter 2. You can also find useful information at the US Department of Agriculture online MyPyramid (formerly known as the Food Guide Pyramid). By using an interactive system available online (www.mypyramid.gov), you can personalize the government's dietary guidelines for your own child. Even if you veer away from American Academy of Pediatrics (AAP) guidelines or MyPyramid recommendations from time to time, don't become discouraged. On occasion, you'll run into unexpected disruptions that keep you from making a trip to the supermarket or spending time preparing meals in the kitchen. Everyone becomes sidetracked from time to time, so don't expect perfection. Even so, never lose sight of your objective, and stay headed in the right direction. Your goal should be to provide your child with a healthy, varied diet as regularly as possible, with choices from each food group. An occasional slipup—perhaps when, by necessity, the family is eating on the run—isn't going to undermine your toddler's good health.

Now, what about portion sizes? They should be appropriate for your child's age. For a toddler, a serving size should be approximately one fourth of the portion appropriate for an adult. A serving of vegetables for a toddler would be about 1 to 2 tablespoons. For meat, a serving might be about the size of their palm.

Picky Eaters

Although toddlers are beginning to develop food preferences, they also can be unpredictable about what they may want for a particular meal on a specific day. Their favorite food one day will end up being thrown on the floor the next. The food that they had spit out, day after day, will unexpectedly turn into the one they can't get enough of.

Picky eating is often the norm for toddlers. For weeks, they may eat 1 or 2 preferred foods—and nothing else. They may eat a big breakfast or lunch and then show no interest in eating much of anything else the rest of the day. Don't become exasperated with this kind of behavior. Just make healthy food choices available to your youngster, and acknowledge that his appetite or food preferences today may be quite different than yesterday's or tomorrow's. That's just the way toddlers are.

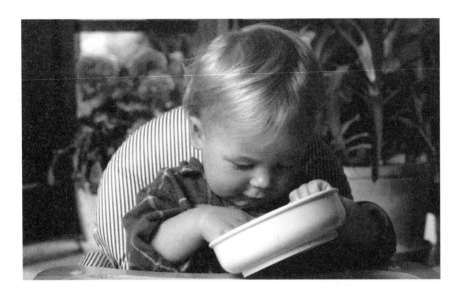

With time, your child's appetite and eating behaviors will reach some equilibrium. He'll find something he likes in a variety of healthy foods without much or any prompting from you. In the meantime, try dealing with picky eaters by giving them finger foods or table foods that they can feed to themselves. Just make sure these are healthy food choices such as slices of banana or small pieces of toast. Also avoid finger foods that could cause choking. Children don't fully develop the grinding motion involved in chewing until they're about 4 years old, so stick with foods that are small and easy to chew and avoid those that might be swallowed whole and get stuck in your toddler's windpipe.

That means avoiding

- Raw carrots
- Raw celery
- Whole grapes
- Peanuts and other nuts
- Large sections of hot dogs
- Raw cherries with pits
- Round, hard candy

Even when your toddler is feeding himself, it's a good idea to sit with him while he eats. He's also old enough to join the rest of the family in eating at the dinner table. Use these family meals to model the healthy eating that you want your child to adopt for the rest of his life.

Sample Daily Menu for a 2-Year-Old

This menu shows a typical day of healthy eating for a 2-year-old who weighs about 27 pounds. (For additional options for snacks, see page 165.)

Breakfast

- Cereal ($1/_2$ cup, iron-fortified) or 1 egg
- Citrus or tomato juice ($1/_2$ cup) or cantaloupe or strawberries ($1/_3$ cup)
- Toast ($1/_2$ slice)
- Margarine or butter ($1/_2$ teaspoon)
- Jelly (1 teaspoon)
- Two-percent milk ($3/_4$ cup)

Snack

- Crackers (4)
- Cream cheese (1 oz) (1 oz = 2 tablespoons)
- Juice ($1/_2$ cup)

Lunch

- Sandwich ($1/_2$): Whole wheat bread (1 slice), meat (1 oz or 1 slice)
- Margarine or butter (1 teaspoon) or salad dressing (2 teaspoons)
- 2 tablespoons dark-yellow or dark-green vegetables
- Low-fat oatmeal cookie (1 small)
- Two-percent milk ($1/_2$ cup)

(continued on page 164)

Snack

- Apple ($^1/_2$, sliced), grapes ($^1/_3$ cup, sliced), or orange ($^1/_2$)
- Two-percent milk ($^1/_2$ cup)

Dinner

- Meat (2 oz) (2 oz is about the size of your child's palm.)
- Vegetable (2 tablespoons)
- Pasta, rice, or potato ($^1/_3$ cup)
- Margarine or butter (1 teaspoon) or salad dressing (2 teaspoons)
- Two-percent milk ($^1/_2$ cup)

Preventing Choking

Your toddler's chewing and swallowing abilities aren't fully developed until 8 years of age. That means that she's more susceptible to choking and should be supervised while eating, whether at home or a child care setting. Here are some suggestions to reduce your toddler's risk of choking.

- Your toddler should be seated when eating. While sitting down, she's more likely to focus on the food in front of her and in her mouth.
- Don't allow your toddler to eat while in a moving car. As the car swerves or brakes, it could change the position of food in your toddler's mouth, leading to a choking episode.
- Round, firm foods such as hot dogs, whole grapes, and apple chunks are common choking dangers. Until your youngster is 4 years old, do not feed her any round, firm food unless it is chopped completely.
- Remind your toddler not to speak with food in her mouth. She should swallow food before talking.

What About Dietary Fat?

If you're worried that your toddler is overweight or concerned that he might become obese at some time in the future (perhaps because obesity runs in your family), you might already be thinking about cutting down on the amount of dietary fat he consumes. As we mentioned earlier, you should think again.

Here's the bottom line: *in the first 2 years of life, you need to avoid placing any restrictions on the amount of fat your child consumes.*

Your toddler actually needs fat in his diet to ensure proper growth and brain development, and those first few years of life are particularly crucial. Dietary fat serves a number of other important functions as well, including providing energy and promoting wound healing. It also helps your child absorb certain vitamins.

How much fat is enough? During his first 2 years, about half of his calories should come from fat. Then after age 2 years, you can modify his diet gradually until his dietary fat makes up about one third of his caloric intake.

Selecting Snacks

For your toddler, snacking should be part of his daily diet. Here are examples of some appropriate snacks for this age group.

- Fresh fruits: bananas, apples, peaches, sliced pears, nectarines, plums (sliced and pitted), strawberries
- Vegetables: peas (mashed for safety), potatoes (cooked and diced), steamed broccoli and cauliflower, green beans (well cooked and diced), yams (cooked and diced)

- Meat and protein: fish (fresh or canned tuna), peanut butter (smooth, spread thin on a cracker or bread)
- Dairy foods: milk, yogurt (fresh or frozen), cheese (grated or diced), cottage cheese
- Breads and cereals: whole wheat bread, soft bagels (cut into tiny pieces), crackers, dry cereal, rice cakes, no-salt pretzels

The Active Toddler

Physical activity is important for children of all ages. Of course, it may seem that your own toddler gets all the exercise he needs as he's constantly on the move from sunup to bedtime. He's crawling, walking, learning to run and jump, climbing onto and down from furniture without help, and kicking a ball or pulling toys behind him while walking.

By 2 to 3 years of age, your child's physical activity will move to even more challenging levels. As his coordination keeps improving, he'll be able to walk up and down stairs. He'll run easily and start learning to pedal a tricycle. With his short attention span, he may be moving from one activity to the next, almost minute by minute, keeping you on the run just to stay up with him.

We can't overemphasize how important this active play is. To encourage it in your toddler, you should be discouraging him from watching TV. The AAP believes strongly that children up to 2 years should not be watching any TV, choosing instead to participate in supervised physical activity outdoors and indoors. Encourage them to play with siblings or other children their own age. When planning family activities, make them as active as possible.

You can also promote physical activity by using the stroller judiciously. When you're out for a walk, don't automatically sit your toddler in the stroller for the entire trip. Let him get out and walk beside you if that's what he wants to do.

If your toddler attends child care, find out how active he is there. In too many child care settings, the TV set and not the kids gets a real workout during the day. Safety should also be a big concern while your toddler is in the child care setting whether he's playing or eating. Request that he always be seated while being fed, rather than running around with food in his mouth on which he could end up choking.

WORKSHEET TO TAKE TO YOUR PEDIATRICIAN
#18: THE TODDLER YEARS

Use your visits to the pediatrician's office to get all your questions answered and concerns resolved. Use the following assessment to help you identify those areas you'd like to discuss with your doctor.

Where Is Your Child Now?
How is your toddler's overall health? _____

Nutrition
Does your toddler seem to have a normal appetite? _____

Does your toddler eat a variety of foods? _____

Does your toddler eat meals and snacks at regular times? _____

What is your toddler eating in child care?

_____

_____

What is your toddler eating at friends' and/or relatives' houses?

_____

_____

Activity/Inactivity
Is your toddler physically active, particularly when compared with other children the same age? _____

Does your toddler watch TV? _____

If so, how many hours does your toddler watch on a typical day? _____

Does your toddler have safe, supervised places to play? _____

Behavior
Does your toddler have any behaviors that concern you?

_____

_____

Are family members working together on good nutrition and activity habits?

_____

What Is Going Well?
Using the previous information, list areas that are going well relative to your child's

Health

_____

Nutrition

_____

Activity/inactivity

_____

Behavior

_____

What Problems Exist?
What childhood health issues are raising concerns?

_____

_____

_____

Do you have any worries about your toddler's nutrition?

_____

_____

_____

Do you have any concerns about your toddler's level of activity/inactivity?

_____

_____

_____

What (if any) behaviors are making it difficult to make good nutrition and activity changes?

_____

_____

_____

(Worksheet continued on page 170)

What Changes Do You Need to Make and How Can You Make Them?
What obstacles are preventing you from making changes to resolve the problems you've identified?

_____

_____

_____

_____

With your pediatrician's help, identify ways in which you can resolve these problems, step by step. Begin by singling out one problem, then determine and list ways in which you can start attacking this concern. Next, work to turn the problem into a success.

_____

_____

_____

_____

Use the following space to note any additional issues or questions that you'd like to discuss with your pediatrician about your toddler's nutrition, physical activity, and other issues relevant to keeping your toddler healthy. Take this list with you to your pediatrician's office.

_____

_____

_____

_____

10
The Preschool Years

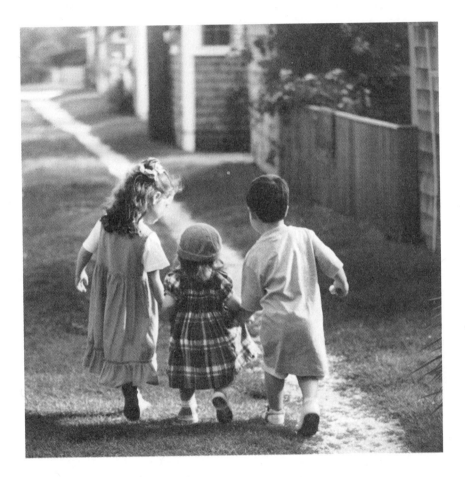

Your child's body has undergone significant changes since the day you brought her home from the hospital. By now, as she moves through her preschool years, your child's baby fat has been replaced by increases in muscle development, accompanied by a slimming of her arms and legs and a tapering of her upper body. Many children at this age still have a small potbelly or pear shape. Some youngsters of this age appear skinny, and their parents often worry that their children are undernourished or perhaps have illnesses that make them look thin.

Then there's the other end of the spectrum, where parents worry about something quite different. Their children are heavier than their playmates. These kids may be eating larger meals and snacking more often than their peers. They might be watching more hours of television and spending fewer hours being physically active.

The fact is that children come in many shapes and sizes. With their weights in mind, most kids fall within the normal range, although in recent years, more parents than ever are being told by their pediatricians that their youngsters are overweight. Your child's doctor has been charting her height and weight since she was an infant, typically during every office visit in the first 2 years of life and then about once a year after 2 years. Your pediatrician can show you your child's growth chart and tell you whether she has gained too much weight. The doctor may calculate your child's body mass index (BMI), which after age 2 years is a good indicator of whether she is overweight. If your child's BMI is above the 95th percentile for her age, she has a weight problem. (For a description of BMI, see page xxix.)

Amid the current epidemic of obesity, the preschool years are a time when a growing number of youngsters are first identified as overweight. If your child has received this diagnosis, you and your family need to follow your pediatrician's guidance on how to begin the journey toward successfully managing this condition. Your doctor's recommendations will probably be very similar to those in this book, including guidelines for healthier eating and increased physical activity. Your doctor will monitor the strategies and efforts that your family begins adopting in the months and years ahead, making sure that your child is progressing in a healthy way.

What Is Your Child Eating?

If your preschool-aged child is overweight, you'll probably need to make some adjustments in her diet. Rather than focusing primarily on cutting down on calories, for example, most of your attention should be placed on ensuring that she eats a variety of healthy foods each day. Make certain that she's eating balanced meals served in portions that are appropriate for her age. (Restricting calories carries potential risks in a growing child, so you should do so only under the supervision of your pediatrician.)

Your entire family should show their support and join the effort to reshape your household's nutrition. To help you make optimal food selections for your family, refer frequently to the information in Chapter 2, as well as the government's MyPyramid Web site, www.mypyramid.gov, and the American Academy of Pediatrics (AAP) book *Guide to Your Child's Nutrition*, keeping in mind that these are guides, not prescriptions. Your overweight child and the rest of the family should try to balance their eating on a daily basis. However, if your child or others in the family have a day when she's eaten too much or has had too little physical activity, take a step back and say to yourself, "This was today; tomorrow's a new day." Variations in eating patterns and activity are inevitable.

As you move your child and the rest of the family in the direction of healthier eating, you'll also find that preschool youngsters have already developed clear food preferences, but that these preferences may change from one day to the next. Kids might gobble up a particular food one day, perhaps even ask for seconds—and then refuse to eat the same food the following day. They may insist on eating a specific food for several days in a row, and then push it away on the days that follow. Don't make this kind of behavior a point of contention; it's quite normal in preschoolers. Just be sure that your children are being given healthy choices at every meal. As a parent, your job is to provide your youngster with good nutritional options in the proper portions each day, then let your child decide whether to eat some or all of it, depending on how hungry she is or her preferences on that particular day. Don't stop serving vegetables, for example, just because your child pushes them away during one or several meals. If you back away from preparing and giving her vegetables or anything else that might not be one of her favorites, you could eventually end up with a child who eats only peanut butter and french fries!

In choosing portion sizes, start by giving your overweight youngster modestly sized servings, and increase them only if she asks (and if your pediatrician approves, if your youngster is on a weight-loss program). Younger children in your family should be served smaller portion sizes than older siblings and parents. Meals and snacks should be structured, meaning that you should provide your youngster with appropriate portions and choices at appropriate times that fall in line with the family meal schedule. This type of structured eating helps children manage their hunger and reduces the likelihood of inappropriate snacking. On the other hand, if your child snacks or grazes all day long, she'll probably cherry-pick her favorite foods during regular meals, rather than eating foods from all food groups. (For guidance on proper portion sizes, refer to page 28 in Chapter 2, which provides examples of serving sizes for 4- to 6-year-olds.)

Reducing Dietary Fat

Up to the time your child is 2 to 3 years old, you should have made no effort to reduce the amount of fat in her diet. That's because the brain in particular relies on dietary fat for proper growth and development in these earliest years of life. Now that she's a preschooler, you can start to gradually reduce the levels of fat that your child consumes. By serving her lower fat meals, you'll help keep her weight under control and lower her risk of heart disease and other chronic illnesses later in life.

Between the ages of 4 and 5 years, you should reach a level where your child is getting fewer calories from fat (rather than the 50% she had been consuming up to 2 years). Once she reaches this lower target of fat intake, it will coincide with the recommendations made for most adults and older children, so your entire family can now be eating the same diet. At this time, most of your family's calories (about 55% to 60%) should come from carbohydrates, with more modest amounts of fat and protein.

What kind of fat-reducing changes should you be making?

- Switch your preschooler from whole milk to skim or 2% milk (which the rest of the family may already be consuming). She should be drinking 2 cups a day of fat-free or low-fat milk (or equivalent milk products).
- Select grilled or broiled fish or lean meats.
- Serve cheese only in modest portions.
- Give your child whole fruit to meet her recommended fruit intake, limiting fruit juice consumption to no more that 4 to 6 oz per day (from ages 1 to 6 years). Remember, this is 100% juice, not juice drinks.
- For snacks, rely on low-fat choices like pretzels, fresh fruit, air-popped popcorn, or fat-free yogurt.
- When preparing food, use cooking methods like steaming, broiling, and roasting that don't require fat during cooking, or use only a small amount of olive oil or nonstick spray.

Remember, meals don't have to be elaborate to be nutritious and support a weight-control effort. You can prepare a healthy meal in minutes—a turkey sandwich, serving of peas or green beans, piece of fruit, and glass of milk. In fact, many young children prefer simple foods, so on days when you're pressed for time, there's no need to spend 45 minutes in the kitchen preparing dinner.

When it comes to snacks, don't leave food out on the kitchen counter that your overweight child and siblings can grab whenever they want. Limit snacks to 2 per day, and provide your kids with healthy choices. Instead of candy or chips, offer them fruit, a slice of low-fat cheese, finger sandwiches, reduced-fat or natural peanut butter on crackers, 1 serving of dry cereal, a couple of low-fat

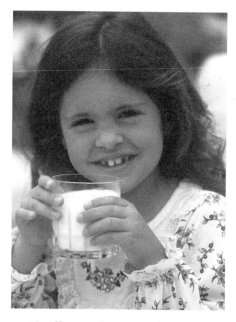

oatmeal cookies, or a bran muffin. Desserts like cake and ice cream are fine occasionally, but not as a daily treat. By limiting, but not eliminating, the consumption of sweets, you'll not only ensure that your family is eating a more nutritious diet today, but you'll lay the groundwork for healthy eating habits that can last for the rest of your children's lives.

Finally, cut down on your family's visits to fast-food restaurants. Unless you're very selective about what your children eat there, they can end up consuming more fat and calories than they do at home, sabotaging your efforts at promoting good nutrition and effective weight management. When you go, make an effort to choose healthy options like fruit and milk rather than fries and soda.

Television and Your Child's Diet

The TV should be off when your child is eating. There is plenty of unconscious eating that can take place in front of the TV, with children snacking their way from one program to the next. Preoccupied with the TV, they'll often eat long beyond when they're full. The result? Weight gain.

Your child should have her meals at the dining room table, eating with other family members as often as possible. Mealtime should be

Sample Daily Menu for Preschoolers

This typical menu was designed for a 4-year-old weighing about 36 pounds.

Breakfast

- One-half cup of 2% milk
- One-half cup of cereal
- Four to 6 oz of citrus or tomato juice or $1/_2$ cup of cantaloupe or strawberries

Snack

- One-half cup of 2% milk
- One-half cup of banana
- One slice of whole wheat bread
- One teaspoon of margarine (or butter)
- One teaspoon of jelly

Lunch

- One-half cup of 2% milk
- One sandwich—2 slices of whole wheat bread, 1 teaspoon of margarine (or butter) or 2 teaspoons of salad dressing, and 1 oz of meat or cheese
- One-fourth cup of dark-yellow or dark-green vegetable

Snack

- One teaspoon of peanut butter or 1 slice of low-fat cheese
- One slice of whole wheat bread or 5 crackers

Dinner

- One-half cup of 2% milk
- Two oz or about $1/_4$ cup of meat, fish, or chicken
- One-half cup of pasta, rice, or potato
- One-half cup of vegetables
- One teaspoon of margarine (or butter) or 2 teaspoons of salad dressing

a valuable time for family conversation and sharing the day's experiences, without the diversion of the TV.

There's another important downside to excessive TV watching. Hour after hour, your child will be exposed to a steady stream of TV advertising, much of it for high-sugar, high-fat foods. Many of these ads are directed specifically at children and promote processed foods that are low in fiber and protein. More often than not, impressionable children will tell their parents that they must have the particular type of cereal or sweet that they've seen on TV, making it even harder to keep kids traveling on the road to healthier eating. Studies have shown that children who watch a lot of TV have a greater likelihood of becoming obese, and the commercials targeted at children are one of the reasons why.

Even if your child doesn't eat in front of the TV, you still need to restrict her TV watching. The AAP advises a daily limit not to exceed 1 to 2 hours of TV viewing, including time spent playing computer and video games.

What if Your Child Becomes Angry?

When you're making changes in your family's lifestyle that may involve everything from what you put on the dining room table to how often you allow the TV set to be turned on, don't be surprised if your preschooler and siblings are annoyed (or worse) at times. If you're going to help your youngster manage her weight, you can expect some groaning and complaining and even some outbursts of anger. Whenever you make changes like those described in this book, whether they are fewer trips to fast-food restaurants or more physical activities for the *entire* family, there will probably be some grumbling. If you're not careful, you might be tempted to give in to this anger by letting your child have a doughnut or turning the TV back on. But that approach will undermine your other efforts to get her weight under control.

To reduce the likelihood that your child will react with anger, make sure that the changes you're making are applied to your entire family. If you serve your overweight child different foods than others at the dining room table, she'll feel singled out and isolated. If everyone is eating a healthy dish of fruit as a dessert, however, she's much more likely to accept it as the new way of doing things.

When angry outbursts do occur, it's good to already have a plan in place to deal with them effectively. Talk with the other adults in the home and agree in advance on how you all will respond to these temper tantrums about your family's lifestyle changes. Here are some suggestions.

- Stay calm. Don't react to your child's anger by becoming irritated yourself. That will only put you and your youngster on a collision course and escalate the difference of opinion rather than resolve it. A lot of parents take their children's outbursts personally and end up lashing out themselves, which is never helpful.

- Give your child a time-out. Perhaps have her sit in a chair for a few minutes and tell her, "When you can talk nicely, you can come back into the family room." Time-outs work if you're consistent and remain calm.

- Stay the course. Never lose sight of the fact that you're making these long-term changes for the health of your family, and explain that to your child. Say something like, "We all want to be healthy, and just like all of us buckle our seat belts to keep us safe in the car, we're going to eat a little differently, too, so we stay healthy." Don't give in to her insistence that she turn on the TV or play more video games, and don't make deals (avoid statements like, "OK, just this once I'll let you watch cartoons until dinnertime, but then you can't ask me to do it again tomorrow"). If you hold your ground, your child will realize that all of her complaining is a waste of energy, and these episodes are likely to decrease in frequency.

Preventing Choking

Your child's chewing and swallowing abilities aren't fully developed until 8 years of age. That means that she's more susceptible to choking and should be supervised while eating, whether at home or a child care setting. Here are some suggestions to reduce your preschooler's risk of choking.

- Your child should be seated when eating. While sitting down, she's more likely to focus on the food in front of her and in her mouth.
- Don't allow your child to eat while in a moving car. As the car swerves or brakes, it could change the position of food in your child's mouth, leading to a choking episode.
- Round, firm foods such as hot dogs, whole grapes, and apple chunks are common choking dangers. Until your youngster is 4 years old, do not feed her any round, firm food unless it is chopped completely.
- Remind your child not to speak with food in her mouth. She should swallow food before talking.

- If you decide to reward your child for good behavior and willingness to follow the new family rules, don't use food as that reward. Positive attention, praise, or a hug are often all the reward she needs. Perhaps give her a sticker or read an extra bedtime story.

Increasing Physical Activity

Your preschool-aged child may seem like she has an endless supply of energy, enough to keep her active for most of the day and night. Too often, that energy never gets used. Because preschoolers frequently spend hours a day in front of the TV, their high energy levels go to waste, giving rise to an increased risk of becoming overweight. Today's children are 4 times less active in their day-to-day lives than their grandparents were. That kind of statistic is troubling and calls for some parental intervention.

As we've emphasized throughout this book, you need to do more than modify your child's eating habits to help promote weight loss. Another effective way of combating obesity is to keep your child physically active. During a child's preschool years, you should encourage free play as much as possible, which will help her develop motor skills. At this age, improving coordination will make your child more agile and allow her to participate in games and activities with greater skill. Even more important than turning to highly structured activities, find safe and adult-supervised opportunities where your child has time for unstructured play, which is crucial to development. In a real sense, play is a child's work, and it is key to helping her grow physically as well as socially, emotionally, and intellectually.

Watch your child during these times of spontaneous play and you'll see how her motor skills are improving. Rather than darting aimlessly from one activity to another, she'll be much more interested in (and capable of) playing tag with other kids or riding her tricycle for long periods. She'll become adept at catching a bounced ball and throwing a ball overhand. She'll run, skip, hop, jump, and walk up and down stairs without holding onto a rail. She'll perform somersaults and climb on playground apparatuses. She'll also develop creativity and problem-solving abilities, learn to cooperate with playmates, and discover the world around her.

Provide your child with age-appropriate play equipment, from balls to plastic bats, to make exercise fun, but let her choose exactly what to play with at any given time. When you're planning family time, schedule family physical activities whenever possible, whether going for a bicycle or tricycle ride on the nearby bike path, kicking a soccer ball back and forth in the local park, or playing catch in the backyard. Remember, parents are important role models for physical activity.

Keep in mind that your preschooler's physical skills are developing far faster than her good judgment. Her playtime needs to be supervised, particularly to keep her from dangerous situations like chasing a ball into the street.

Child Care Guidance

If your preschooler spends time in a child care setting, she should be physically active for much of that time. Safety must be the first priority. Does the child care facility provide safe outdoor and indoor play areas for your youngster and other kids? Is your child always supervised, not only during play periods, but while eating? Is the food your child is being served there compatible with the nutritional goals you're trying to reach at home? (If not, ask for changes in the lunch or snacks or pack food that your child can bring with her.) Are your child and others seated while eating or running around with food like raw carrots in their hands and mouths, increasing the risk of choking?

Particularly when your child is enrolled in a new child care setting that you're not fully familiar with, it's a good idea to drop in unannounced at various times of the day to make sure that your youngster is getting the kind of care being promised. If the kids are huddled around the TV set rather than actively playing or outdoors unsupervised near a heavily traveled street, it's time for some changes, including finding a new child care center if appropriate adjustments can't be made.

If your preschooler is overweight and on a weight maintenance eating plan, make sure the child care providers know what dietary restrictions your youngster has. They need to be partners in this effort toward normalizing your child's weight, and if they're feeding your child high-fat snacks, insist on some healthier alternatives.

WORKSHEET TO TAKE TO YOUR PEDIATRICIAN
#19: THE PRESCHOOL YEARS

Use this questionnaire to help you determine how your preschool-aged child is progressing and identify any concerns you may want to raise with your pediatrician during your next office visit.

How Is Your Child Currently Doing?
How is your preschooler's overall health? _____

Does your preschooler seem to have an abnormal appetite? _____

What foods does your child routinely refuse to eat?

_____

Does your preschooler demand certain foods? _____

Does your child eat meals and snacks at regular times? _____

Is your child physically active, particularly when compared with other children the same age? _____

What activities does your preschooler participate in?

_____

Does your preschooler watch TV? If so, how many hours does he or she watch on a typical day (weekday and weekends)? _____

Does your child have a TV in his or her bedroom? _____

Does your preschooler watch TV during meals daily? _____

What is Going Well?
Using the previous information, list areas that are going well relative to your child's health.

_____

_____

_____

What steps have you taken to lower the levels of dietary fat in your youngster's diet?

_____

_____

How many 6 oz glasses of milk (2%/1%/whole) does your preschool-aged child drink daily?

_____

What Problems Exist?
What childhood health issues are raising concerns?

_____

Do you have any worries about your child's appetite?

_____

_____

Is your child a picky eater? _____

Is your child a picky eater in certain food groups? _____

How often does your family eat at fast-food restaurants in a typical week? _____

What other nutrition-related issues concern you?

_____

Is it difficult to get your child to be physically active? _____

What Changes Need to Be Made?
What obstacles are preventing you from resolving the issues that you've identified?

_____

What steps could you begin taking to ensure that your child eats healthier, more balanced meals?

_____

_____

_____

What measures could you use to lower the levels of dietary fat in your youngster's diet?

_____

_____

(Worksheet continued on page 188)

How can you integrate more activity into your child's life?

_____

_____

_____

_____

Choose a single problem you'd like to deal with and identify and list solutions to it. Next, begin to implement these strategies and record your successes here. Also, identify who can support you and your child in these efforts (for example, spouse, relatives).

_____

_____

_____

_____

Based on your answers in this assessment, use the following space to write down questions and concerns that you'd like to raise with your pediatrician about your preschooler's nutrition, physical activity, and other issues relevant to his or her health. Take this list with you to your next doctor's visit.

_____

_____

_____

_____

11

The School-age Years

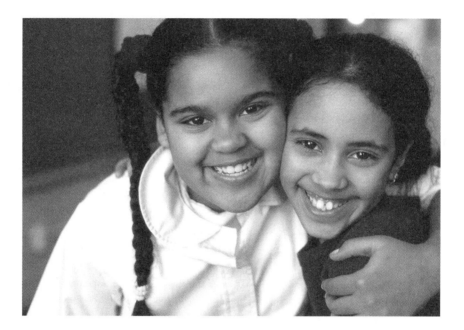

E very stage of your child's life presents challenges for you and your youngster, including the school-age years. During this time in his life, your child will be adjusting to new educational and social settings, interacting with more children than ever before, and making many new friends. He'll also be developing new academic skills and increasing his knowledge of the world. All the while, he'll be relying on you for advice and guidance.

If your child is overweight, both of you have some additional challenges. In many families, when children have been heavy since their preschool years, their parents expect—or at least hope—that this weight problem will finally resolve itself as young bodies grow and mature from the ages of 6 through 12 years. That often doesn't happen. Shortcomings in nutrition and inadequate physical activity that began early in life often continue throughout childhood, unless a conscious effort is made to change course. For example, even though there are many ways for your school-aged child to be physically active, the TV and computer games may be winning the battle for your child's time and attention. As a result, his weight might continue to climb.

At each visit to your pediatrician's office, the doctor calculates your child's body mass index (BMI) (see page xxix) and can tell you whether he's exceeding the normal range on standard growth charts. During the school-age years, children gain weight at a steady rate to match their growth; as they approach puberty, those increases in weight will accelerate. If your pediatrician has raised some red flags, cautioning you about excessive weight gain, you need to take it seriously. Overweight children are much more likely to become obese adults, which will place them at risk for serious chronic disorders such as heart disease and diabetes. However, with the support of your pediatrician, this is a time when you and your child can make changes that direct him along the proper path toward better health. As your pediatrician may tell you, these are very important years for helping your child adopt healthy eating and activity habits that can last a lifetime. By taking steps like serving your youngster appropriate foods in the right amounts and encouraging him to be physically active every day, any weight concerns that exist now will become less of a problem as he gradually moves toward the "normal" range on your pediatrician's growth chart.

Eating for Good Health

What was your initial reaction when you realized that your child needed to control his weight? In that situation, many parents find themselves thinking, "I've got to put him on a diet." After all, in a culture in which thinness seems to be the name of the game and Americans just can't get their fill of diet books, you might instinctively think that the solution rests with the latest weight-loss fad, even though these diets are rarely designed with growing children or good nutrition in mind.

No matter what some diet gurus proclaim, calorie counting and exercising to the point of fatigue are *not* the answer, particularly for children. In fact, restricting calories in a growing child could pose risks to his health. You shouldn't do so unless your pediatrician recommends and supervises those efforts.

So what's the answer? As we've emphasized throughout this book, consistently good nutrition, meal after meal, is a foundation for a healthy childhood. Rather than becoming preoccupied with weight-loss goals, you should focus instead on a wholesome lifestyle for everyone in your family, no matter what each member weighs. Establish some structure to your family's eating—3 well-thought-out meals and 2 snacks a day. If you take steps to minimize the junk food in your family's diet, eliminate sugared beverages like soft drinks, pay attention to portion sizes, and add some physical activity to the mix, your heavy child *will* grow up to have a healthy weight.

In preparing foods high in nutritional value, build the family meals around selections like

- Fresh fruits and vegetables
- Whole-grain cereals and bread
- Low-fat or nonfat dairy products like milk, yogurt, and cheeses
- Lean and skinless meats including chicken, turkey, fish, and lean hamburger

The basics of good nutrition really aren't that complicated. It means choosing low-fat turkey bologna instead of beef, or preparing a grilled chicken sandwich instead of a high-fat cheeseburger. Refer to Chapter 2, as well as the government's online MyPyramid (www.mypyramid.gov), if you need a refresher course on the types of foods that should be part of your child's diet each day. Portion sizes at this age should be less than that of an adult-sized serving. Remember that when you're in the kitchen, choose cooking methods that involve a minimal amount of fat, relying primarily on broiling, roasting, and steaming.

During these middle years of childhood, there are plenty of obstacles that can trip up your well-intentioned efforts at keeping your family eating right. In the mornings, as you're rushing to get your child off to school, are there days when he doesn't have the time to sit down for a nourishing breakfast? At school, does he sometimes make poor choices in the cafeteria or from vending machines?

As a parent, part of your responsibility is to find solutions for any stumbling blocks that arise. If the school cafeteria doesn't offer many healthy choices or your child cannot be convinced to purchase healthy options (and in many elementary and middle schools, only one lunch entrée is provided), pack a healthy lunch for your child each day. You might prepare a turkey sandwich on multigrain or pita bread. A peanut butter and jelly sandwich is fine, too. There are plenty of good selections, but stay away from pastrami, salami, and other high-fat lunch meats. Add a piece of fruit to your child's lunch sack and perhaps a bag of pretzels. Pack a small water bottle for him, or give him money to buy low-fat milk in the cafeteria.

Once your child gets home from school, he might head straight for the cupboard or refrigerator and look for something to munch on. Have some healthy snacks for him to choose from—raw vegetables with nonfat dip, fresh fruit, whole-grain crackers, air-popped popcorn, unsalted pretzels, or baked tortillas with salsa. Keep the ice cream, cookies, and cakes out of reach—or better yet, out of the house altogether (reserve them for special occasions). If you don't limit access to snack foods like these, you're unfairly setting your child up for a losing battle against weight gain.

Meanwhile, stay alert for other potential stumbling blocks to healthy eating. For example, your school-aged child may sometimes exchange food with friends, giving up the sandwich and fruit that you've packed for him and trading them for a bag of potato chips. After school, if he's spending time at a playmate's home, he might be snacking there on candy rather than an apple. In short, even if you've done a good job of educating your child on making nutritious food choices, he'll face plenty of temptations, almost on a daily basis. (See "'It's Not Fair!'" on page 196.)

Also remember that you're a role model in this process, so make healthy food choices for yourself as well as the rest of the family. Even though school-aged children are busier than ever, make an effort to find time for family meals as often as possible. When all of you sit down at the dining room table together, it's a perfect opportunity for every family member to describe his or her day and the family to grow closer.

Making Sense of Childhood Eating Behaviors

During these years from ages 6 through 12, children need good nutrition to keep growing normally. As they approach adolescence, most girls experience increases in their growth rate between the ages of 10 and 12 years, while boys will begin their greatest growth spurts about 2 years later. Some parents worry that throughout the school-age years, there seems to be no rhyme or reason to their children's appetite. One day, they may eat everything in sight, while on other days, they might turn into such a finicky eater that you'd expect their stomachs to be growling throughout the day.

In most cases, these kinds of unpredictable eating patterns shouldn't concern you. During this time of life, children should be gaining about 4 to 7 pounds a year, and as long as your pediatrician tells you that your child is growing normally and his weight gains are fine, don't worry about the number on the scale. Instead, keep your focus on serving a variety of healthy foods. Expect his appetite to vary, sometimes considerably, from one day to the next.

At the same time, children in this age group eat for a lot of reasons besides hunger. Even when they complain that they're starving, hunger may not be the reason why they want something to eat. They

"It's Not Fair!"

On average, school-aged children eat at least one meal a day away from home. Often, that meal is at school or friends' homes, and you don't always know what and how much your youngster is eating. No wonder most parents have heard their children griping that friends or classmates have some privilege, experience, or food that they don't.

It can be frustrating, but stay in control as much as possible. Never lose sight of the fact that you're in charge of your home environment. You are the person who decides what food is in your house and when and how much food will be available for your child there. You're the one who makes decisions in supermarkets. You're the one who stocks the kitchen cupboards and eliminates undesirable foods or saves them for special occasions. At the same time, it's important to provide all your children with age-appropriate explanations of why your family is making nutritional changes. Keep in mind that while an 11-year-old can comprehend much more about the need to improve the food choices on your dinner table than a 6-year-old, most children understand when you tell them that "our entire family is making changes so we can be as healthy as possible."

Now, what can you do when your school-aged child is away from home? As you've already read on page 195, you'll lose some control over what he eats when he spends time at friends' houses. He might be able to choose soft drinks instead of milk there, or cookies rather than an apple or orange. At a fast-food restaurant with friends, he might feel peer pressure to choose a supersized burger and fries rather than a smaller hamburger and salad. But you can enlist the help of the parents of your child's friends—ask for their support in keeping unhealthy snacks away from your child, making it easier for your youngster to make better choices. The same goes for other adults with whom your child spends time, including child care providers and grandparents.

Sure, your child might complain, "Everyone else has cookies in their lunch bags. Why do you give me an orange instead?" Or you may hear the common refrain, "It's not fair!"

Well, he's right—it may not seem fair. Remind him, "We're trying to eat better in our family because we care about our health." If your child is old enough to understand, try accentuating the positive. For example, "You're a good student—you inherited that from our family. You also know that our family has trouble with weight, and we have to take care of that so we can stay as healthy as possible."

As these changes are made, let your child feel some sense of control over the situation. Let him make choices among a number of healthy alternatives.

Encourage him to lend a hand in the kitchen, preparing a meal now and then. Explain why milk is a better selection than soda and why a pear is healthier than a candy bar. Remind your child that he can have the cookies or chips that he craves on occasion, although not as an everyday treat, At the same time, introduce him to healthier alternatives that he may develop a taste for, such as low-fat baked tortilla chips rather than higher fat potato chips.

could be upset or tired and relying on food for comfort. For some children, eating may merely be a habit—for example, they're used to gobbling up snack foods anytime they're watching TV or playing video games. When your youngster says that he's hungry and it's not a regular meal or snack time, try to determine what's really going on and whether food might be serving some other purpose. Then problem solve. If your child seems to be bored, for example, help him find an activity that will keep him occupied doing something productive and steer him away from food. Distracting your child's hunger with a fun, physical activity is one way of achieving 2 goals.

The Hazards of Sneaking Food

Imagine thinking that your overweight child is making all the right nutritional choices, and then discovering a bag of potato chips or cookies in his dresser drawer. Or just when you think that he's sticking to the rules, you discover that the snack foods that were on a high shelf in the kitchen cupboard have "mysteriously" vanished. In fact, plenty of school-aged children sneak food, often believing (or at least hoping) that they'll never get caught. Quite often, they seem surprised when they're confronted about their behavior. In fact, they may deny it at first before finally admitting that they've been doing it for weeks or months.

In Chapter 6, you read about the perils of sneaking food, which can be common in school-aged youngsters. Children of this age may sneak for a variety of reasons. Perhaps eating can ease the stress they're experiencing over upcoming examinations or because they're being teased or bullied at school. Maybe they just want to feel a greater sense of control over their environments.

When you become aware of sneaking behaviors, keep your own disappointment or anger in check. Let your child know that you've discovered that he's been hoarding food, and talk with him about why he's doing it. Remind him about the family goal of healthier eating, and offer to help him find other strategies to meet his emotional needs aside from food. Suggest positive ways for him to respond when he feels that he absolutely has to eat something, even when it's not time for a regular meal or snack. For example, he can

- Ride his bicycle.
- Go for a walk with you.
- Kick a soccer ball with a friend.
- Read a book.
- Paint a picture.
- Exercise with a workout video.
- Finish a crossword puzzle.

On page 110, we described setting up a reward system and giving your child privileges when he asks for food rather than sneaking it. He might earn points that he can accumulate for rewards like renting a DVD or video game. Talk about these rewards in advance, and stick to them. For many children, this system can be very effective in minimizing sneaking. Never punish a child for eating the wrong foods, even if this occurs soon after you've explicitly instructed your child not to do so. Removing privileges may be hard to resist, but resist them. In a year or two your child may become more naturally interested in controlling his unhealthy eating impulses. Do not allow negative strategies this year to jeopardize future possibilities of success.

Making Fitness a Way of Life

Some school-aged children can't wait to get home from school, stake out a place on the couch, and spend the rest of the afternoon and evening watching TV. Physical activity is just not on their radar screens, at least not by choice.

Not surprisingly, children who fit this profile may be on a slippery slope to a life of obesity. There are a lot of them. Several years ago, when a group of children 6 to 12 years old participated in programs of the President's Council on Physical Fitness, only 50% of girls and 64% of boys could walk or run a mile in less than 10 minutes. If that same study were conducted today, when the obesity epidemic seems to be gaining momentum, those statistics might be even more troubling.

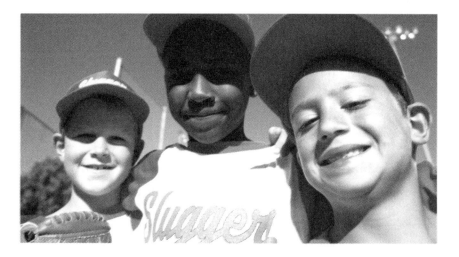

During your child's school-age years, your goal should be not only to get your child moving, but to turn exercise into a lifelong habit. There are plenty of opportunities for your child to keep active.

In most communities, children in this age group can choose to get involved in a number of organized sports, including Little League, youth soccer, a martial arts class, or community basketball, hockey, or football leagues. Team sports are fun and the perfect fit for many youngsters, and they can help them manage their weight.

However, group activities like these aren't for everyone. Some obese children feel self-conscious about participating in team sports and are much more comfortable getting their exercise in unstructured settings. For them, free play on the playground, ice skating, in-line skating, bowling, or even running through sprinklers is good exercise. Let your child choose something that he finds enjoyable, and once he discovers it, encourage him to make it a regular part of life. At the same time, limit TV watching or time spent on the computer or playing video games to no more than 1 to 2 hours a day. Studies have shown that the more time children devote to watching TV, the more likely they are to consume foods like pizza, salty snacks, and soda that contribute to weight gain.

What if your child insists that he doesn't want to do any physical activity? Explain that it's important and might even be fun to find a new activity. Try to find activities that fit the family's budget and time commitments and have him choose among several alternatives. Some children might prefer to go with a friend or parent. Be creative and emphasize participation, not competition. To help your school-aged youngster become physically active, recruit the entire family to participate. Let your overweight child know that all of you, parents and siblings alike, are in his corner, and even if he has rarely exercised before, he can start now with the entire family's support. Go for family bike rides (with everyone wearing a helmet). Swim together at the Y. Take brisk walks. Learn to cross-country ski. Sign up for golf lessons.

You can even do activities of daily living together, such as household chores. Spend a Saturday afternoon cleaning the house or raking leaves. No matter what you choose, regular activity not only burns calories, but also strengthens your child's cardiovascular system, builds strong bones and muscles, and increases flexibility. It can also diffuse stress, help him learn teamwork and sportsmanship, boost his self-esteem, and improve his overall sense of well-being.

For further guidance on physical activity, see Chapter 3.

Where the American Academy of Pediatrics Stands

Throughout this book, we've emphasized the concerns that the American Academy of Pediatrics (AAP) has with children watching TV, particularly in excessive amounts. When it comes to children's programming, the primary goal of the networks is to market the products of advertisers—from toys to junk food—to children. Younger children, in particular, including those in the early elementary school years, cannot distinguish between programs and the commercials that surround them, nor do they fully understand that the intent of advertising is to get them (and their parents) to buy products in supermarkets and toy stores.

The AAP strongly supports improvements in the overall quality of children's programming and encourages parents to limit the amount of time that their kids spend in front of the TV.

The Role of Your Pediatrician

During your child's school-age years, he may see your pediatrician for routine well-child examinations about every 1 to 2 years. If your youngster is overweight, you may need to schedule appointments more often. Your pediatrician can regularly calculate your youngster's BMI. The doctor can help guide your family toward better nutrition and more physical activity as well as help you troubleshoot if you're having difficulties in one health-related area or another.

WORKSHEET TO TAKE TO YOUR PEDIATRICIAN
#20: THE SCHOOL-AGE YEARS

Before your next visit to the pediatrician's office, fill in this questionnaire and take it with you. It will help your doctor see how your school-aged child is progressing, and it can identify problem areas that need some intervention.

Use this visit to the pediatrician's office to get all your questions answered and concerns resolved.

How Is Your Child Currently Doing?
How is your school-aged child's overall health? _____

Does your school-aged child have a regular appetite? _____

Does your child eat meals and snacks at regular times? _____

Does your child eat a variety of foods? _____

Is your child physically active? _____

What activities does your child participate in?

_____

Does your youngster watch TV? _____

Does your child have a TV in his or her own bedroom? _____

If so, how many hours does your child watch on a typical day? _____

What Is Going Well?
To gain some perspective, use the previous information to list key areas that are going well relative to your child's health.

_____

_____

_____

What Problems Exist?
What specific concerns do you have about your school-aged child's overall health?

_____

_____

_____

Do you have any worries about your child's appetite?

_____

Is your child a picky eater? _____

Does your child sometimes refuse to eat or demand certain (unhealthy) foods? _____

Do other family members create a home environment that unnecessarily tempts your child? (For example, does a parent really like having premium ice cream in the freezer? Do older sibling always keeps the TV on? Does a grandparent show love with home-baked goods? Does a parent place small amounts of fruit in the bottom shelf of the refrigerator and bulk purchases of brownies on the eye-level shelf?)

_____

_____

In a typical day, how many meals does your child eat away from home? _____

How often does your family eat at fast-food restaurants in a typical week? _____

Does your child watch TV while eating, and does he or she often overeat in the process? _____

What other nutrition-related issues concern you?

_____

Is it difficult to get your child to be physically active? _____

What Changes Need to Be Made and How Will You Make Them?
What obstacles are preventing you from resolving the issues that you've identified?

_____

_____

What steps could you be taking to ensure that your child eats healthier, more balanced meals?

_____

_____

What measures could you use to lower the levels of dietary fat in your youngster's diet?

_____

_____

How can you integrate more activity into your child's life?

_____

_____

(Worksheet continued on page 206)

Choose a single problem you'd like to begin dealing with and identify and list solutions to it. Next, begin to implement these strategies and record your successes here. Also, identify who can support you in these efforts (for example, a spouse, relatives).

_____

_____

_____

Based on your answers in this assessment, use the following space to write down questions and concerns you'd like to raise with your pediatrician about your school-aged child's nutrition, physical activity, and other issues relevant to health. Take this list with you to your next doctor's visit.

_____

_____

_____

_____

12

The Adolescent Years

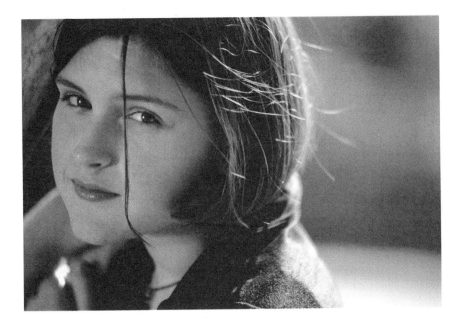

*I*f there's a teenager in your family, you don't need to be reminded
about the many challenges of parenting an adolescent, guiding her
from childhood into adulthood. If your teenager is also overweight
and the issue of obesity has been added to the mix of challenges, it
might seem as though your parenting skills are constantly being
put to the test.

Perhaps you've already spoken to your pediatrician about just how
high the stakes are for your adolescent and her present and future
health. An obese teenager not only faces health risks today such as
diabetes, liver disease, lipid problems, hypertension, and sleep apnea,
but also has about an 80% chance of becoming an obese adult. If
she's heavy as she enters adulthood, she'll have a much greater
likelihood of developing these diseases as a young adult.

To complicate matters, you probably feel that you have less control than ever over the factors that are contributing to your teenager's
excess weight. After all, she's probably spending less time at home
than she used to, limiting your opportunities to prepare meals and
encourage her to exercise. No wonder so many parents in your situation assume that the weight issue is largely beyond their influence.
At times, you might find yourself thinking, "She eats so many meals
away from home…how can I possibly have an effect anymore?"

That's certainly not the case.

Yes, your teenager is much more independent than she was 5 or
10 years ago, but she's not yet an adult. You're still a very important
person in her life, and it's essential that you stay connected. It's true

that your involvement may no longer be the 24/7 hands-on role that you played in the past, but don't minimize the effect you can still have on the choices she makes. You need to stay an active participant in her life and be there to help her build the skills and nurture the behaviors that promote healthy eating and regular physical activity.

Your Changing Role

Your teenager is a different person than she once was. As an adolescent, she may not be capable of assuming adult responsibilities quite yet. As she has grown and matured, she's now much more able to understand the implications and consequences of being overweight. You can reason with her much more effectively. As a result, you should address the issue of obesity differently than you once did.

Here's an example of how your approach might change. When your teenager was younger, did you sometimes use rewards to motivate her to make health-promoting changes? As a school-aged child, did she respond to your offers of stickers or a few more minutes of TV watching if, in return, she agreed to spend an hour playing on the playground with friends? As effective as that strategy may have been, it probably won't work anymore. Yes, perhaps a younger adolescent (13 or 14 years old) may be willing to change her behavior if you offer her small amounts of money in return (face it—stickers just aren't going to work at this age!). Yet by the time she's 15 years or older, you need to shift gears. When her weight is concerned, appeal to her sense of reason. Help her understand the social and health consequences of being obese in a world that's often unfriendly to heavy people.

For instance, if your youngster is 15 years old, you might ask her, "What do you think will happen if you just keep gaining weight?"

Don't expect her to respond by saying, "Well, I might get diabetes or high blood pressure, and I don't want that to happen." However, she might open up and begin talking about the way overweight students are teased at school. Or she might describe how hard it can be for heavy kids to keep up with their peers in physical education classes. Like all teenagers, she's also probably conscious of and concerned about her body image, and she knows what classmates might be saying about the way she looks. Those kinds of situations might motivate her to change in ways that will allow her to effectively attack the problem of excess weight.

In the process, let your adolescent know that despite her growing independence, you're still her parent and you'll still be there when she needs you. You might say, "Let's continue to work on your weight together. We can still go on family hikes on the weekends. We can still go on bike rides. I'll continue to prepare nutritious meals when you're home, and there'll be plenty of healthy choices in the refrigerator for snacking. I'm not willing to completely back away just because you can make a lot more decisions on your own now."

At the same time, let your teenager know, "I'm always available to talk with you about any problems you may be having with food away from home—maybe bad choices you're making in the school cafeteria or at friends' houses." Make suggestions, gently offer advice, but also give your teenager some space to make choices on her own, and let her know that you trust her to make good ones. Sure, there will be times when she doesn't make the best decisions, but at her age, putting more control in her hands works better than saying, "Here's what you need to do—turn off the TV and go outside right now!" or "I don't care where your friends like to go—you've got to stop eating at fast-food restaurants!"

Keep the dialogue open with your youngster. Ask questions like, "What's been the hardest part about managing your weight this week?" "What can I do to help?" "What can we think of together that will keep you moving in the right direction?"

Explain to your teenager that, in a sense, you've become something akin to her coach. Remind her that even the most elite athletes need coaches, and it isn't a sign of weakness or failure. Don't offer advice at every turn, or she's liable to shut the door without even listening. Just let her know that you're available to talk and give guidance when she wants it. By all means, create a home environment that's conducive to success.

The bottom line is that your role is changing, and that means posing some questions to yourself, too. For example, are you asking your teenager to make changes in her eating or activity level that you're not doing yourself? Are you sabotaging her efforts to eat healthy by keeping junk food in the pantry or baking holiday cookies and leaving them out where she can't help but be tempted? Are you framing your comments to your youngster in a supportive manner? For instance, rather than asking, "Why are you so lazy when it comes to exercising?" you could say, "Why don't we get the entire family to go play tennis this afternoon?"

One additional thought: Even though your teenager is much more capable of taking the weight issue into her own hands, she can still use all the support that's offered. So you and your other family members should join forces to become your teenager's most loyal support team. Let your adolescent know that the entire family will provide what she needs to help her make wise decisions about her weight. Sometimes, teenagers may act as though their friends are much more important to them than family. You and the rest of your family will continue to be much more indispensable to her than she's sometimes willing to admit.

Nourishing Your Growing Teenager

Ask the average adolescent to describe her perfect meal, and she's liable to say, "A double cheeseburger with large fries," or maybe, "Pepperoni pizza—as many slices as I can fit on my plate."

For a teenager with a weight problem, however, those may not be the optimal choices, as popular as they may be. No matter how your own teenager would describe her ideal meal, there's no doubt that nutrition is crucial at this time of life. She's going through puberty and growing rapidly and, particularly if she's heavy, she needs to become conscientious about eating a healthy diet.

If you need a refresher course on balanced, nutritious meals, refer back to Chapter 2. Here are just a couple key points to keep in mind.

- Teenagers need to eat foods from all the major food groups (see page 23) and rely more often on lower fat choices. That means grilled chicken sandwiches more often than a cheeseburger and consuming meals with vegetables and fruits as well as pasta, rice, and a variety of other foods.

- Serving sizes for teenagers should be about the same as they are for adults. Rather than putting serving dishes on the dining room table and letting family members help themselves, prepare everyone's plate away from the table to keep from tempting your overweight adolescent to help herself to seconds—and thirds.

As you use the information in Chapter 2 as a guide, there are some obstacles that your teenager may face when trying to eat in ways that support effective weight management. Following are some examples.

Skipping meals. Adolescents are renowned for skipping meals—most often, breakfast and/or lunch—and this can throw their entire nutritional programs off-kilter. According to a recent poll, about one half of all boys and girls aged 9 to 15 years said that they didn't eat breakfast on school mornings. Your teenager may tell you that she prefers to sleep a little later, even if it means leaving for school on an empty stomach.

Even if your adolescent believes that those extra minutes of sleep are just too precious to sacrifice, there are ways to still keep her well nourished. Why not spend a few minutes in the evening preparing a breakfast-to-go for the following day? Perhaps you can slice a bagel that can be quickly toasted in the morning (use peanut butter rather than cream cheese as a spread). Hard-boil an egg that can be eaten in the car. Put some nuts and raisins in a plastic bag for her to nibble on. Let her feast on a container of yogurt or an apple. All of these choices may be enough to tide her over until she's able to sit down for a well-balanced meal later in the day.

Snacking. For the average teenager, snacking seems to be a way of life. In fact, one third of the caloric intake of adolescents comes from snacks. Yet too often, their preference of snack foods is a little suspect. Given the choice, many teenagers would rather grab a handful of potato chips than grapes.

Keep in mind, however, that when it's time for a snack (which, for many adolescents, is most of the time), they'll reach for what's available. For that reason, make an effort to keep your refrigerator and pantry stocked with healthy snacks. That means choosing foods like low-fat cheeses, nonfat frozen yogurt, applesauce, air-popped popcorn, and baked potato chips.

Eating away from home. Because teenagers eat many of their meals outside the home, adult caregivers aren't there to keep an eye on what they're putting on their plates. Not surprisingly, some of their choices fall short of what they should be.

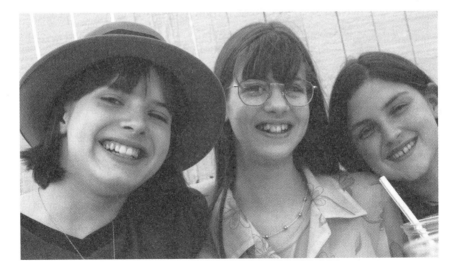

At school, some adolescents will settle for a stop at the vending machine at lunch and consume a bag of cookies and a soft drink before their next classes. If they're eating at a fast-food restaurant or a pizza shop with friends, they may decide that fitting in with their peers is more important than making healthy food selections.

When your teenager is away from home, you can't reasonably ask her to avoid fast-food restaurants, particularly when that's where her friends go on Saturday night. But you can ask her something like, "Can you think of anything you could order besides a large hamburger, large fries, and a shake?" Remind her that it doesn't have to be an all-or-nothing proposition, and if she's open to suggestions, perhaps you can guide her toward making healthier decisions ("How about choosing a smaller burger or a chicken sandwich, plus a salad with low-fat dressing?") If she's going out for pizza with friends, remind her that while she can certainly have a slice of pizza, why not balance it with a salad? She might also develop a taste for thin-crust vegetarian pizza instead of thick-crust pepperoni pizza with double cheese.

Remember, this is a learning process, and you can't expect your teenager to always make healthy choices. Over time, she'll get better at it. Also remind her that when she's out with friends, she doesn't have to eat the entire time. Often, just hanging out with her buddies is enough. For example, ask your adolescent, "Can you suggest something else to do with your friends besides going to a restaurant? Maybe you could go bowling or to the batting cages?" On the other hand, she might tell you, "I'm going to feel funny if I don't eat something when all my friends are ordering food." She may be right, but she can still be more selective in the food she buys and puts on her plate.

The lure of fad diets. Sometimes, it seems as though teenaged girls talk as much about diets as about boys. Particularly if they're preoccupied with their weight (and what adolescent girl isn't?), they can probably hardly wait to share the newest quick-fix eating plan they've found, latching onto one crazy diet or another with little attention paid to how poor its nutritional value might be. One month, they might be trying a low-carbohydrate diet, then a high-carbohydrate diet the next. Or they'll become hooked on a grapefruit diet one week and a fruit-free diet the following week. They probably won't stay on any of them for very long, but as they hopscotch from one to another, good nutrition may fall by the wayside. These diets are usually too restrictive and too unhealthy. With weight loss in mind, they won't work over the long run, either.

Endless hunger pangs. Does it seem like your teenager is *always* hungry? Since she entered and began moving through puberty, have you noticed that the refrigerator and kitchen cupboard doors are getting a real workout, hour after hour, day after day? Does it seem like shortly after a trip to the supermarket, it's time to go back because the cupboards are becoming bare again?

As part of adolescence, your child's appetite may be soaring off the charts as her need for calories escalates to support normal growth spurts. Nevertheless, despite her constant craving for food, you and your youngster don't have to give up the battle against her weight problem.

Here's a basic principle to keep in mind—as long as you're providing your adolescent with well-balanced nutrition and high-quality foods, and she's eating 3 reasonably sized meals per day plus 2 snacks, her weight should be just fine. If she's still telling you with regularity that she's absolutely famished, and if it's also a time when she's growing, feed her, but make sure you're giving her nutritious food, not a couple of candy bars. When you stick to healthy foods from the major food groups, her weight will take care of itself.

Wielding Your Influence

If your teenager is like most others, she probably doesn't shop much in grocery stores. She leaves that to you, which allows you to remain the major influence on the foods she consumes in your home.

Whenever possible, encourage the family to have meals together. The fact is that families who eat together tend to have healthier diets than those whose members prepare something only for themselves or eat away from home a lot. A study at Harvard Medical School evaluating the diets of 16,000 boys and girls aged 9 to 14 years found that those who frequently ate with their parents were 1.5 times more likely to eat the recommended number of servings of fruits and vegetables each day. Not only will your adolescent probably get better nutrition during these family meals, but you can also serve as a role model for the way she should be eating, even when she's not at home.

When Eating Gets Out of Control

If your overweight teenager's attempts at sensible weight loss don't seem to be working, and she moves from one fad diet to another with nothing to show for it but a lot of anguish and frustration, she might ultimately decide to join the ranks of many other adolescents by resorting to the desperate lifestyle of an eating disorder like bulimia nervosa. As their preoccupation with weight and body image intensifies, these teenagers may start bingeing on food (often high-calorie junk food), consuming thousands of calories at a sitting, with seemingly no control over what they're doing. Once a bingeing episode has run its course, which could take an hour or two (or sometimes more), they purge themselves by self-induced vomiting or abusing laxatives or diuretics.

For most bulimics, these bingeing-and-purging cycles repeat themselves day after day. These teenagers eat emotionally, even when they're not hungry, typically trying to compensate for or cope with low self-esteem and feelings of inadequacy. They usually feel guilty about and disgusted by what they're doing and often hide food in their dresser drawers or closets. They may be-come depressed or experience mood swings, and despite symptoms like swollen glands in their necks and erosion of their tooth enamel (which is associated with vomiting), they can't stop this cycle of emotional eating.

More than 10 million Americans have one type of eating disorder or another—not only bingeing and purging to avoid gaining weight, but also under-eating or self-starvation (anorexia nervosa), as well as gorging on food without any purging involved in it. Although these eating problems affect primarily girls and women in their teens and twenties, some boys have these disorders as well. They can go undetected for years, with bulimic teenagers often planning their bingeing-and-purging episodes when no one else is home.

(continued on page 220)

As a parent, be on the lookout for behaviors that lead you to suspect bulimia in your adolescent. Bulimia is a complex disorder—you can't assume that your teenager is going to outgrow it or that you can put a stop to the problem simply by telling her to quit. When the problem finally comes out in the open, become a good and nonjudgmental listener. To support her recovery, you also need to seek professional help for her, and the earlier this intervention takes place, the better. Contact your pediatrician, who will probably refer you to a specialist or treatment facility in this field. Your teenager will probably receive behavioral therapy (psychotherapy), nutritional counseling, and medications such as antidepressants to help her in the recovery process.

Teens, Diet Pills, and Surgery

Anyone who has tried to lose weight and keep it off, whether adolescents or adults, knows that it isn't easy. It takes commitment, perseverance, and plenty of patience.

In a society that values the quick fix, it's not surprising that some obese teenagers are turning to diet pills as the magic bullet to deliver them from the hard work of eating right and exercising regularly. In search of an easy solution, adolescents are asking their parents (and pediatricians) for weight-loss prescription drugs with increasing frequency. Or they're going to pharmacies on their own and buying over-the-counter diet pills that promise to melt away the pounds with no effort at all.

Your own overweight teenager might be tempted to turn to these drugs, but it's unwise for her to do so. Let your adolescent know that there's no over-the-counter weight-loss drug that's been proven safe and effective for teenagers. Orlistat, a prescription weight-loss drug that blocks fat absorption in the intestine and has been approved by the Food and Drug Administration for children older than 12 years, is only useful in a few teens who meet strict criteria. This drug needs to be used under physician supervision to monitor the teen's nutrition and side effects of the drug. Weight control requires an effort over many months and even years, and none of the over-the-counter drugs were developed for long-term use.

Here's where you need to assert your parental authority. *Your teenager should not take diet pills.* There are safer ways to lose weight, and they're described throughout this book.

Now, what about weight-loss surgery? A small number of centers in the United States are performing gastric-bypass and similar forms of surgery in extremely obese adolescents. Any surgical procedure carries risks, so these procedures should only be done in centers doing ongoing research into the long-term risks and benefits. Even though these operations can have dramatic weight-loss benefits, your teenager will still have to improve the way she eats and exercises in the aftermath of the surgery.

Talk to your pediatrician about the pros and cons of these operations, and if the doctor feels your adolescent is a candidate for the procedure, the pediatrician may refer you to a surgeon for an evaluation.

Breaking a Sweat for Weight Loss

Many children seem to be in constant motion in their early years. All of that activity often comes to an end in adolescence, as the time and opportunities for physical activity begin to wane. At many middle and high schools, physical education programs have been curtailed or completely eliminated. Add to that the demands of after-school activities such as music lessons and school plays, part-time jobs, homework, and the availability of TV, video games, and computers, and many adolescents complain that there simply isn't time to be active.

Throughout this book, we've stressed the importance of getting your overweight child off the couch and finding ways for her to become active. Chapter 3 had plenty of suggestions to help your child get moving, from encouraging her to walk on the treadmill to going in-line skating to signing up for a karate class. Nearly every teenager can find some form of activity that she enjoys and is willing to do regularly, whether it's throwing a ball with a neighborhood friend or joining an evening basketball league at the Boys & Girls Club. Don't forget the lifetime sports that your teenager can develop a love for that can last for decades, including golf, tennis, skating, and skiing.

What if your overweight adolescent resists doing any kind of activity? Don't give up hope. If she seems glued to the TV or computer, ask her, "What else can you do besides watch TV?" If she says, "I don't know," you might say, "Let's figure it out together." Sometimes, you can get her interested by saying, "Let's both sign up for an exercise class at the Y—I'll take the adult class, and you take the one for teens."

Frankly, any form of movement is better than letting your youngster sit in front of the TV all afternoon. Encourage her to get out of the house, even if doing so doesn't involve an overtly physical activity. Encourage her to volunteer at the senior center, or maybe she can join the choir at church. She can get a part-time job at the community recreation center, helping organize games for younger kids. Then see if there's a way to build some exercise into those seemingly sedentary activities. When you drop her off for choir practice, can she get out of the car at the far end of the parking lot so she has to walk a hundred yards to the church entrance? If she's working at the recreation center, can she fit some walking into her required tasks?

By the way, even if you often hear the complaint, "I don't have time to exercise," your teenager may actually have more time than she thinks. There are probably 15 or 20 minutes during her afternoon or evening when she's sitting in front of the computer and could shift gears and use some of that sedentary time for physical activity.

WORKSHEET TO TAKE TO YOUR PEDIATRICIAN
#21: THE ADOLESCENT YEARS

Spend a few minutes filling out the following questionnaire and take it with you on your next visit to the pediatrician's office. Your doctor can help you and your teenager solve any difficulties that have arisen in your adolescent's efforts to manage his or her weight effectively.

How Is Your Adolescent Currently Doing?
How is your teenager's overall health? _____

Does your teenager have a normal appetite? _____

Does your adolescent eat meals and snacks at regular times? _____

Does your teenager eat a variety of foods? _____

Is your teenager physically active? _____

What activities does your teenager participate in?

_____

Does your youngster watch TV? _____

If so, how many hours does your teenager watch on a typical day? _____

How much time does your adolescent spend using the computer or playing video games? _____

What Is Going Well?
To gain perspective, use the previous information to list key areas that are going well relative to your child's health.

_____

_____

_____

What Problems Exist?
What specific worries and concerns do you have about your teenager's
overall health?

_____

_____

Do you have any worries about your adolescent's appetite and/or what he or
she is eating?

_____

_____

Is your teenager a picky eater? _____

Does your youngster sometimes refuse to eat or demand certain
unhealthy foods? _____

In a typical day, how many meals does your teenager eat away
from home? _____

How often does your family eat at fast-food restaurants in a typical
week? _____

Does your adolescent watch TV while eating, and often overeat in
the process? _____

What other nutrition-related issues concern you?

_____

_____

Is it difficult to get your teenager to be physically active? _____

What Changes Need to Be Made and How Will You Make Them?
What obstacles are preventing you from resolving the issues that you've
identified?

_____

_____

_____

(Worksheet continued on page 226)

What steps could be taken to ensure that your teenager eats healthier, more balanced meals?

_____

_____

_____

What measures could you use to lower the levels of dietary fat in your youngster's diet?

_____

_____

How can you integrate more activity (and less TV and computer games) into your teenager's life?

_____

_____

Choose a single problem you'd like to begin dealing with and identify and list solutions to it. Next, begin to implement these strategies and record your successes here. Also, identify who can support you in these efforts (for example, a spouse, relatives).

_____

_____

_____

_____

Based on your answers in this assessment, use the following space to write down questions and concerns you'd like to raise with your pediatrician about your adolescent's nutrition, physical activity, and other issues relevant to his or her health. Take this list with you to your next doctor's visit.

_____

_____

_____

_____

13
When Problems Arise

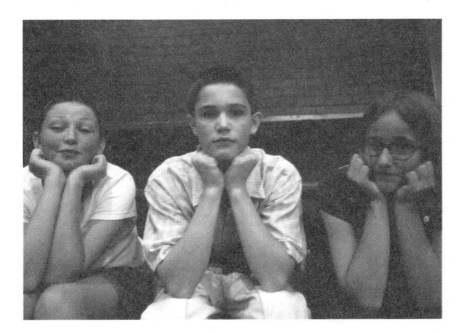

If you've ever tried to lose a few excess pounds yourself, you know that the journey toward weight loss is filled with challenges. It's no different when your child walks along that same path toward a healthier life. No matter how conscientious you and your child are, problems will arise and obstacles will surface. In this chapter, we'll describe some common hurdles—and solutions—that you might have already confronted or could encounter in the weeks and months ahead.

So often, the questions or statements posed by parents are in the format of, "Yes…but." For example, "*Yes*, my child should exercise more, *but* there's just no time," or "*Yes*, I'd like to get the cookies out of our house, *but* what should I tell the other kids who still want cookies here?"

All of the following parental questions or statements are presented in this format. The solutions may help you troubleshoot problems that arise in your own household.

"Yes, I'd like to give my kids more fruits and vegetables, but fresh produce is too expensive!"

Fresh fruits and vegetables may be more affordable than you think. Particularly if you buy them when they're in season, they'll be much more reasonably priced than at other times of the year. Also, compare the costs of produce to other foods that you may already be buying for your child. For example, processed foods—from cookies to potato chips—are not only more expensive, but they certainly aren't as nutritious as fresh fruits and vegetables.

A number of studies have confirmed that fresh produce is more affordable than you might think. In 2004, the US Department of Agriculture analyzed and released data from household food purchases made in 1999, including multiple types of fruits and vegetables. The researchers concluded that the average American can purchase 4 servings of vegetables and 3 servings of fruits for just 64 cents a day. If this figure were adjusted to today's costs, the price might be an average of less than a dollar a day. No matter how you analyze the numbers, that's a great deal.

By the way, the same study found that two thirds of all fresh fruits and more than half of all fresh vegetables are less costly than processed versions of the same produce.

"Yes, I'd prefer to feed a variety of vegetables to my overweight child, but he absolutely hates vegetables. The only 'vegetables' he'll eat are french fries. That's it!"

As a parent, your job is to provide your child with well-balanced meals, including a variety of vegetables. Once the food is on the plate in front of him, he may choose whether to eat it. Sure, it can be frustrating when kids push the plate away and refuse to even try something new, but be persistent. The good news is that over time, most children will develop a taste for enough healthy foods—even some vegetables—to be eating a balanced diet.

Some children may be more agreeable to consuming vegetables if you ask them to help you in the kitchen while you're preparing meals. They may be more receptive if you add vegetables to a pasta dish or put them in soups or meat loaf. Some youngsters prefer raw vegetables over cooked, and they'll often snack on cherry tomatoes or cut-up vegetables with yogurt dip. When eating in restaurants, accompany children on trips through the salad bar; expose them to vegetables they may never have tried at home.

Meanwhile, continue to serve as a role model. If your child sees you eating vegetables, he's more likely to try them. Have him get used to the idea that vegetables are part of every lunch and dinner. Remember your child will need to have at least 1 serving of fruits and vegetables with every meal and snack to meet the recommended 5 servings a day.

"Yes, I know my overweight child shouldn't have dessert with dinner every night or sweetened juices whenever he wants them, but I feel terrible if he complains about feeling deprived."

Don't lose sight of why you're making these dietary changes. As a parent, your child's health must be a top priority, and that may require making some adjustments in what he eats and the amount of physical activity he gets.

Of course, you don't want your youngster to feel deprived, and there's no need for you to completely eliminate his favorite desserts from his life. However, save those treats, like rich ice cream or chocolate chip cookies, for special occasions and serve appropriate portion sizes when you do. At the same time, introduce him to healthier desserts such as a dish of strawberries or a piece of angel food cake. When beverages are concerned, rely more often on low-fat milk or water rather than sugar-laden soft drinks or juices. Before long, he'll stop demanding the high-calorie, high-fat treats that he once craved.

"Yes, I'm willing to get unhealthy foods out of the house, but other adults in the home haven't come onboard yet. They tell me that they've been drinking sugary soft drinks all their lives, and they're not willing to give them up."

If other adults in the home insist on keeping high-fat snacks or high-calorie drinks in the cupboard or refrigerator, those kinds of temptations aren't fair to your child. To support your youngster's efforts to lose weight, it's essential for the entire family to get involved. The family needs to sit down and discuss the implications of continuing to live a lifestyle of poor eating choices. If the others still can't be convinced of the potential consequences of doing their own things, perhaps your pediatrician can talk to them. With your youngster's health at stake, your pediatrician may be able to motivate the others to give some ground. If they need to have sugary soft drinks, ask them to indulge at work and leave those kinds of snacks out of the house.

"Yes, my own mother seems to understand how important it is for my child to lose weight, but she still thinks it's a grandmother's prerogative to give my child candy whenever we visit. How can I convince her to get rid of that candy dish?"

The answer to this question is not much different than the previous one about others in the home having an attachment to soft drinks. You need to talk to your child's grandmother about the health risks your youngster faces unless he eats more nutritiously, one meal and one snack after another. As accustomed as grandma may be to baking cookies when the grandchildren visit, you can probably appeal to her strong desire to give your child the best possible chance of living a healthy life. Refer back to Chapter 2, and let grandma know about the nutritious food choices she can have available for the next family visit.

"Yes, I realize that when the family goes out to dinner, we should stay away from fast-food restaurants most of the time, but whenever we drive by one of those places, my child pleads with me to stop."

It's fine to eat at fast-food restaurants once in a while. Because of their high-fat fare, though, don't make it a habit. Try and encourage lower fat options at fast-food restaurants.

When you visit these types of restaurants, order carefully for the family, finding choices to keep your child happy without sabotaging his healthier eating efforts. Whenever possible, for example, select a grilled chicken sandwich without any dressing for your youngster. If he insists on a hamburger, choose the smaller size, not the supersized double burger that looks like it could feed the entire family. Order a salad with low-fat dressing that he can eat as part of his meal.

Rather than overrelying on fast-food restaurants, choose to eat at sit-down family restaurants more frequently and look for healthy options on the menu. Split a dinner between the two of you. You will save money and eat healthier!

"Yes, snacking before bedtime may not be a good idea for my child while he's trying to lose weight, but when I was growing up, my mother always gave us cookies and milk before we went to bed. It's just something that I feel comfortable doing, and it would be hard to do things differently."

Habits may be difficult to break, but for the well-being of your child, you need to make some adjustments. Nothing's inherently wrong with a bedtime snack, but you may need to adjust the kinds of snacks you're offering your youngster.

In general, try to limit the number of snacks to 2 per day. For those late-night munchies, make choices that contribute to overall healthy eating. You might turn to

- Air-popped popcorn rather than high-fat cheeses on crackers
- Frozen yogurt instead of ice cream
- Baked tortilla chips rather than potato chips
- Graham crackers (and milk) instead of chocolate chip cookies
- A piece of fruit rather than sugary cereal

"Yes, I understand that healthy eating is the best way for my child to lose weight, but I sometimes think that he could benefit from a little kick start, and the latest fad diets promise fast results. What's wrong with following one of these diets for a few weeks to get him off to a good start?"

Most people have lost weight at some point in their lives—but then gained it all back. They know that fad diets don't work, at least over the long term, but the alluring promises on magazine covers and book jackets are often too tempting to resist.

Unfortunately, fad diets can be dangerous. They often emphasize a single food or food group, and they can be particularly risky for growing children for whom balanced nutrition is extremely important.

As we've emphasized throughout this book, you need to put your child's health and well-being first. Don't be persuaded by promises of overnight weight loss. Instead, stick with a plan for good nutrition and physical activity like the one described in these pages. Your child's weight loss will be gradual and safe and have the best chance for permanent success.

"Yes, I feel that I can control what my child eats at home, but when he's at child care, I have no control over what the child care provider gives him. He's served whatever the other kids eat."

Express your concerns to the child care staff. Even if the facility serves identical meals to all the children, make some suggestions for fine-tuning the menu in the direction of healthier foods. The staff may turn out to be much more flexible than you expected and might be willing to bend to your requests, perhaps serving your youngster a turkey sandwich and small salad for lunch instead of a hamburger and french fries.

If you're sensing some reluctance on their part, offer to pack your child's lunch and/or snacks to make sure that he's eating foods supportive of the family's commitment to more nutritious eating.

"Yes, I'd love to sign my overweight child up for a fitness program at the Y, but we just can't afford it."

Kids can enjoy the benefits of physical activity without busting the family budget. Play is the major way kids can increase their activity. You don't need costly exercise equipment like treadmills, nor do you have to enroll them in classes with expensive sign-up fees. Outdoor play in a safe area can be a major help to increasing physical activity.

Turn back to Chapter 3, and you'll read about plenty of activities that won't cause financial stress. Walking, for example, is one of the best forms of exercise, and it doesn't require any special equipment, other than a good pair of walking shoes. If the entire family gets involved, your overweight child is more likely to be motivated to walk regularly. In fact, the best forms of physical activity are family activities. Keep them fun, and your child won't feel that he's missing out on the formal program at the Y.

"Yes, my child knows that he needs to become more physically active, but he has so much homework, plus piano lessons after school, and there's just no time for exercise."

So many of today's kids lead very busy lives. It seems as though their planned activities start immediately after school and continue until well after nightfall. If you think about it, there's probably some time in your child's afternoon and evening, even just 15 or 20 minutes, when he could fit in some physical activity.

Remember, activity needs to become a *priority* in your child's life. That means that exercise wins out over video games or surfing the Web almost every time. After school, can he play catch with the neighborhood kids in the park down the block, or work out to an exercise video that you put into the VCR?

Frankly, there aren't too many kids who don't have a few minutes to spare each day for squeezing in some physical activity. Physical activity promotes motor and mental development and is essential for developing coordination.

"Yes, my overweight child should be getting more physical activity, but in our neighborhood, I just don't think it's safe for him to be playing outdoors."

Don't let safety concerns keep your child sedentary. There are plenty of ways for him to stay active other than playing in your front yard or on the neighborhood playground. He can participate in a swimming program at the Boys & Girls Club or join a karate class. He can stay active indoors at home by dancing to his favorite music, spinning a hula hoop, jumping rope, or doing chores like straightening up his room.

"Yes, eating right and being active makes sense, but my teenager has so much weight to lose that we've been talking about weight-loss surgery. Is that something we should consider?"

Although the overwhelming majority of gastric-bypass surgeries are being performed in adults, a relatively small number of teenagers have undergone the procedure. However, this is *major* surgery, and the decision to have the operation should not be made hastily.

Weight-loss surgery is only advisable for extremely overweight adolescents for whom more conservative weight-loss measures haven't worked, particularly if they also have developed serious obesity-related medical conditions such as high blood pressure, diabetes, and sleep apnea.

Your pediatrician can provide an initial assessment of whether your teenager might be a candidate for surgery. If the pediatrician refers you for a consultation to a weight-loss surgeon who performs these procedures, you and your adolescent will meet with the surgeon as well as a number of other specialists, including clinical psychologists and nutritionists. You and your teenager will have the opportunity to discuss the potential benefits of the operation, plus get your questions answered about the complications sometimes associated with the operation like infections, bleeding, and blood clots.

Afterword

*T*his book has given you and your child the tools you need to help
her lose weight and improve her overall health. If she's been strug-
gling with extra pounds for months or years, and if her health has
been suffering in the process, hopefully you've already begun traveling down the path toward making better lifestyle decisions that
can help normalize her body weight.

However, the journey has just started, not only for your overweight
child, but for you, other adults in the home, your other children, and
their grandparents as well. Hopefully, your entire family has decided
to participate in this new adventure. To support your overweight
child, everyone around her needs to be involved in this effort. When
that happens, this new way of living will become the fabric of your
family, and the everyday decisions about eating and physical activity
will become a permanent way of doing things.

Goals for the Future

Since you began reading and implementing the strategies described
in this book, how has your overweight child fared? Perhaps she has
already lost a few pounds and is showing improvements in her overall well-being. Keep in mind, however, that there is no short-term
cure for obesity. Whether a weight problem affects a child or an
adult, it requires a long-term commitment to make the lifestyle
changes that are needed.

In the weeks and months ahead, you and your child should set
some goals to keep the family on track. For example,

Weight goals. In some cases, particularly if your child is younger and still growing, your pediatrician may recommend that your youngster not lose any additional weight at this point, but rather maintain her present weight until her height catches up. As she becomes taller, her body mass index (BMI) will improve as her weight stays the same. By contrast, the goals for a teenager may be different—if your adolescent has already reached her full height, the only way to lower her BMI is to reduce her weight. Even so, losing weight should not be her only goal. In fact, it is not the best way to define success. That leads us to the health goals described as follows.

Health goals. As you read in Chapter 1, obesity can be hazardous to your child's health. It can contribute to many serious health problems, from an increased risk of high blood pressure and diabetes to a greater likelihood of developing asthma and sleep apnea. With your pediatrician's guidance, your child should work to reduce her health risks, perhaps by lowering her cholesterol count and normalizing her blood glucose levels, for example.

To reach these goals, you and your child should place an emphasis on a healthy lifestyle. As you do, the weight loss will take care of itself. As you've already read, we are not recommending typical weight-loss strategies like strict caloric restriction, stringent meal plans, or high-intensity exercise. Instead, you should be encouraging your child to follow the guidelines described throughout the book until they become second nature, including

■ Striving for optimal nutrition by lowering dietary fat intake and increasing the consumption of fruits and vegetables

- Increasing daily physical activity
- Reducing the time spent in front of the TV or computer

Lifestyle modifications like these should become your child's day-to-day goals, beginning in the short term and then lasting a lifetime. Even if your pediatrician has suggested a target weight-loss goal for your child—say, losing 25 pounds to bring her BMI into the normal range—your child's lifestyle choices should not change throughout the process. Even as she approaches and eventually reaches that target weight, she should continue eating the same healthy way and remain physically active. After all, these are the lifestyle adjustments that are bringing your youngster's weight and health back into balance, and it's important for her to keep doing more of the same.

In the process, the entire family needs to adopt a new long-term mindset. In the past, when your overweight child was eating more and gaining weight, that might have been the norm in the family. The key is to turn these lifestyle improvements into your family's new normal. In earlier times, perhaps it was normal for your child to drink 3 sugary soft drinks a day; now, her new normal is to drink water or low-fat milk instead. She's not on a diet—she just has a new normal way of living.

What if Your Child Backslides?

No one's perfect. Everyone slips up from time to time. In adopting the family's new nutritional and activity lifestyle, your overweight child may be doing just fine for weeks, but then she might respond to the stress of final examinations by sneaking food or making inappropriate choices in the school cafeteria. During the holidays, she might overindulge in the traditional desserts that grandma makes. If the entire family has a particularly busy week, all of you may eat out more than usual and regular physical activity may be sacrificed.

When you're talking about adopting a healthy lifestyle over the long term, these kinds of occasional lapses are inevitable. No matter what the reason, when you notice that your child is backsliding, the key is to help her get back on track as soon as possible. Don't allow the slip to turn into a long, downhill slide. Encourage your child so she doesn't become bogged down by frustration or disappointment. In fact, the sooner you intervene, the better her chances are of bouncing back, barely missing a beat. Don't forget to remove easy temptations such as unhealthy snacks.

How can you minimize the risk of future backsliding? Spend some time with your youngster analyzing why the problem occurred. Was the lapse an indication that your child has started making poor choices? Did some short-term distractions take place that could recur? Once she understands the reasons that she stumbled, they're less likely to happen again.

In the meantime, rather than becoming preoccupied with a setback, keep your child focused on everything that she has done right over the past few weeks and months. Remind her of the progress she's made, and encourage her to keep moving forward. Let her know that despite the backsliding, she's still headed in the right direction.

Preparing Plan B

When you least expect it, life events can intervene and derail all of your child's efforts toward a healthier life. Perhaps dad goes into the hospital for surgery; mom decides to go back to school 3 nights a week while also keeping her job during the day; grandma becomes ill, throwing everyone's schedule awry; or you're moving from one house to another, disrupting your usual routines for a couple weeks or more.

However, backsliding during these times can often be avoided if you and your family plan in advance for any events that could sabotage your child's progress toward a healthier life. If you know that a family member's surgery is on the horizon, for example, why not have a fallback plan—plan B—already in place? Rather than letting events that lead to abandoning health-supporting lifestyle changes roll over you, why not decide as a family ahead of time how you're going to deal with them? What steps have worked in the past when disruptions occurred (for example, keeping meals simple and preparing and freezing them ahead of time), and can you implement them again in the future?

Stressful, unexpected events are a part of life, and you need to make sure that they don't undermine the progress your child has already made.

Looking Ahead

Success in weight management isn't going to happen overnight. It's a process, and you should approach it one step at a time. Even when the long-term goals seem challenging, you can and should celebrate the small achievements, one day after another. As your overweight child makes changes in her nutrition and physical activity, they will contribute to her overall success, and you should offer praise for every one of these advances, one week after the next.

Along the way, stay in touch with your pediatrician. The doctor can help you answer the question, "How are we doing?" by monitoring your child's weight and the health improvements that are taking place. The pediatrician also can assist the family in rising above any setbacks. Consider your child's doctor a partner throughout this process.

As you continue to implement the lifestyle strategies described in this book, you should be pleased with the progress your child is making. The key is to keep going.

WORKSHEET TO TAKE TO YOUR PEDIATRICIAN

#22: EVALUATION

To complete this process, let's perform another assessment to help you evaluate how far your overweight child and the entire family have come and what still needs to be done. Answer these questions and talk them over with your pediatrician.

Has your child adopted new health-related behaviors like the strategies described in this book? _____

Is your child eating differently? What modifications in his or her nutrition have been made?

_____

_____

Has your child's activity level changed? _____ What is he or she doing differently now? _____

How many hours a day or week does your child watch TV, play video games, and use the computer? _____

What steps can you take to reduce those numbers?

_____

_____

What problems remain that you and your overweight child would like to tackle in the future?

_____

_____

_____

_____

Index